QUANTUM MEDICINE

A GUIDE TO THE NEW
MEDICINE OF THE 21ST CENTURY

PAUL YANICK, JR.,
PH.D., N.D., C.N.C.

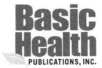

Basic
Health
PUBLICATIONS, INC.

The information contained in this book is based upon the research and personal and professional experiences of the author. It is not intended as a substitute for consulting with your physician or other healthcare provider. Any attempt to diagnose and treat an illness should be done under the direction of a healthcare professional.

The publisher does not advocate the use of any particular healthcare protocol but believes the information in this book should be available to the public. The publisher and author are not responsible for any adverse effects or consequences resulting from the use of the suggestions, preparations, or procedures discussed in this book. Should the reader have any questions concerning the appropriateness of any procedures or preparation mentioned, the author and the publisher strongly suggest consulting a professional healthcare advisor.

Basic Health Publications, Inc.

Library of Congress Cataloging-in-Publication Data

Yanick, Paul.
Quantum medicine : a guide to the new medicine of the 21st century /
Paul Yanick, Jr.

   p. cm.
ISBN 978-1-59120-031-4
1. Detoxification (Health). 2. Naturopathy. 3. Alternative medicine.
I. Title.

RA784.5 .Y36   2003
613—dc21

                 2002154606

Editor: Stephany Evans
Typesetting/Book design: Gary A. Rosenberg
Cover design: Mike Stromberg

Printed in the United States of America

10   9   8   7   6   5   4   3   2   1

Contents

Acknowledgments

There are many people to thank in seeing this book come to fruition: The numerous colleagues who let me try out new ideas, the friends who patiently listened to my brainstorms, the professors and others who led me to deeper knowledge, and the hundreds who offered encouragement and insights. Still, I must single out a precious few for special acknowledgment.

To my wife, Bonnie Lee, for her support, unconditional love, and friendship, and for her organization and management of the many details of making Quantum Medicine a reality. To my children, Heather Rose and Thomas Scott, for their support and love during this time-consuming project.

To my son, Thomas Scott, for his brilliance with computer graphics and word processing in making this book a reality.

To Howard Marr, my long-time and trusted friend, for his many hours of uncompensated hard work in handling the management and educational aspects of the American Academy of Quantum Medicine.

To my parents, whose love and sacrifices made it possible for me to pursue university studies and research. And to my brother Frank for his support and encouragement of my ideas and research efforts.

To Monte Elgarten, M.D., whose medical support of Quantum Medicine and willingness to learn and practice Quantum Medicine made the transition to creating a new medical model easier and less stressful.

To all of you who had any role in assisting me over the years, especially those of you who have adopted the principles of Quantum Medicine and made it your own, thank you. Without you, this book would never have seen the light of day.

A Note to Readers

This guidebook represents decades of scientific research and study in the fields of anatomy, physiology, biochemistry, quantum physics, pharmacology, endocrinology, neurology, nutrition, psychology, anti-aging medicine, and Quantum Medicine. In an effort to make it more accessible to the layperson, I have avoided extremely technical language and omitted thousands of arcane scientific and textbook references. Many of the concepts presented in this book are indisputable facts of life that follow the laws of nature; they are based on natural laws and empirical observations, sound reasoning, and common sense. This book also reflects more than three decades of clinical experience with laboratory-guided observations of the human energy system and nutritional biochemistry in many clinical disorders.

If you have a disease or any other type of health-related problem, you should first consult your physician before attempting to deal with it. This book is not meant to replace a medical examination, and its contents are not meant to diagnose medical conditions, interpret medical symptoms, or render medical advice. It should be used in consultation with your doctor to better understand health problems and their possible range of treatments.

The purpose of this book is to increase nutritional awareness and to educate individuals regarding natural ways to improve their general health and well-being. All readers are encouraged to seek help from doctors who treat people as whole individuals with unique and distinct dietary, exercise, and nutritional needs. The best course of action is for the reader to use common sense and the information in this volume in consultation with a reliable physician to achieve a healthy, fulfilling lifestyle.

Introduction

What if there were a way your body was able to repair a damaged organ or renew and regenerate itself at an accelerated rate? Or a way to regain peak mental and physical performance despite having felt sick and tired for years? Well, there is a way. Today, there are many scientists who believe the secrets of regeneration and healing lie not within costly drugs or expensive medical treatments, but in the body's own genetic world.

The ongoing effort to decode the mysteries of healing in the human body has reached a point where it really now appears possible for us to turn on powerful biological cascades of energy that will speed up renewal and regeneration in our bodies. *Quantum Medicine* presents the extraordinary discoveries that have been made so far in this exciting field, and explains how gaining control of the stress in your life may well be the key to activating your body's own potent medicines for healing, endurance, vitality, and longevity.

As you will learn in this life-transforming book, experiencing the full power of your own healing energies is a matter of your choices and actions. By learning and applying the principles of Quantum Medicine, you can actually accelerate and enhance healing, acquiring greater health and a greater joy in living.

In the United States, we have the world's finest medical care for treating traumatic injury. Yet, when it comes to preventing disease or activating the body's innate healing powers, most American doctors tend to lag behind those in other countries. They simply lack training in Chinese Medicine, Ayurveda, or other time-proven, natural healing methods that seek to reestablish the body's own energetic balance and vitality; they may even lack faith in these modalities.

Many Western pharmaceutical treatments do not cure the condition; they simply block symptoms. When you block a symptom with a drug, you block innate healing. A blocked symptom often rebels by spawning clusters of symp-

1

toms that doctors diagnose as disease. Then they "treat" the disease by just handing out a prescription for every symptom. Shouldn't doctors be educating patients about the causes that underlie their symptoms? I say, yes, they should. Shouldn't they teach their patients how to take greater responsibility for their own health? I believe physicians have a responsibility to do so. That's one reason I have written this book.

In order to facilitate real healing, it is necessary to understand the symptom, coming to grips with whatever is underlying it, or allowing it to express fully what's provoking it. However, mainstream medicine's research remains focused on treating acute conditions rather than on prevention, on caring for the body in such a way that its natural, self-sustaining abilities are enhanced.

Yet it is the general consensus among medical scientists that only about 15 percent of Western medical practices are based on scientific evidence! In fact, a 1997 article appearing in the *Journal of the American Medical Association* reported that the likelihood of finding any specific disease on which to pin a patient's symptoms was less than 2 percent.

Some of the most widely accepted academic teachings, intellectual beliefs, and therapeutic modalities often make the problem of being sick—from any cause—many times worse than it has to be. Hippocrates, the founder of modern medicine, made little use of drugs, believing that they simply interfered with the natural healing processes. He used "fomentations" (medicinal compresses), bathing, diet, and other natural remedies.

Modern medical treatments frequently, in effect, underestimate the body's magnificent intelligence and block its capabilities for self-healing and repair. However, a growing number of frontier scientists, some of them Nobel Laureates, have been assiduously mapping the energetic patterns involved with healing and regeneration. In the past decade, this work has progressed to a point where real solutions are available. These are safe, proven, and time-tested natural therapies that can evoke innate healing, even for the most stubborn cases of a wide spectrum of ailments. These healing breakthroughs involve unleashing the awesome healing power of your entire body, allowing it to function the way it was designed to function, so it can heal itself naturally.

Rather than function like a lifeguard who rescues patients from one health disaster after another in the dangerous surf of today's toxic and stressful environment, doctors of the future will ultimately teach us how to stay healthy by *avoiding* health stressors and by enhancing and nourishing the body's intelligent, life-sustaining quantum energy field (QEF).

The clinical insights of Quantum Medicine go further, all the way down to the inner workings of living cells as they interact with the QEF. Quantum Medicine is demonstrating that the same bodily intelligence that knows how to heal a cut finger or mend a broken bone without your even thinking about it can be enhanced to heal you of almost any ailment. But to accomplish such feats, you will have to work in harmony with your body's anatomy, not against it. You'll need to learn how to nourish it, and how to prevent stress factors from overwhelming it or exhausting its healing energies. You'll need to learn how to empower it to keep you in a state of vibrant health.

Today, the world is on the threshold of a wide spectrum of serious health threats. Dangerous toxins surround us in our "modern" environment. Almost everything we breathe, eat, drink, or wear can contribute to a toxic buildup in our bodies—unless we take charge.

Changes in the environment, in available foods, in nutritional supplements, and even in medicines are all combining to bring about extremely stressful living conditions. According to the National Institute of Environmental Health Sciences, more than *300 billion pounds* of synthetic chemicals were produced, used, and disposed of in the early 1990s. Almost 80,000 chemicals are registered for commercial use, with 2,000 additional new ones being added annually to food, personal-care products, supplements, prescription drugs, household cleaners, and lawn-care products.

Pollutants are being stored, rather than neutralized and excreted out of the body, thereby depleting our bodies' nutrient reserves at an alarming rate. These toxins can diminish our QEFs and immune functions to a mere 50 percent of their original capability. With these critical healing systems functioning at half-potential, it's no wonder that there are so many people suffering with chronic diseases. These foreign chemical invaders go to war with the body's functional unity and healing capacities, and when they win, we acquire an illness. These illnesses force doctors into a maze of uncertainty as they frustratedly label one disorder after another as a "syndrome."

Many experts acknowledge that deadly viral breakouts pose a very real and dangerous threat to our public health. Researchers have identified numerous mutant and novel pathogens that resist currently available antibiotics, that wreak havoc by tricking the immune system into attacking the body. These mutant infections, called *mycoplasmas,* are neither virus nor bacteria, so they often elude detection by conventional laboratory tests. According to one of America's top mycoplasma researchers, Dr. Shyh-Ching Lo, these disease agents contribute to AIDS, cancer, chronic fatigue, Crohn's colitis, type-1 diabetes, multiple sclerosis, Parkinson's disease, Wegener's disease, and collagen-vascular diseases, such as rheumatoid arthritis and Alzheimer's disease. Since 1942, deadly and infectious forms of mycoplasma have even been weaponized in ongoing biological warfare research.

In addition to these threats, in the United States, sepsis (infection) is the most common cause of death in the noncoronary intensive care unit; it's the eleventh leading cause of death overall. Fifty-eight million Americans have high blood pressure, surely exacerbated by today's many forms of stress, with 1.5 million experiencing a heart attack each year. In 1970, one out of fifteen people died of cancer. Today, one in every three Americans dies of cancer.

Our environment can have serious effects on our lives and health. It can undermine the quality of human life and erode human potential. To a degree, we can improve the quality of our personal environment; however, to the degree that we *cannot* change the larger environment, we can at least change the way our bodies respond to it. Preventing the diseases of civilization is a reasonable and attainable health goal. Regular exercise, proper nourishment, and the avoidance of environmental stressors are fundamental ways to regain a sense of self-control in our lives, keeping us physically and mentally fit, and emotionally and spiritually centered.

The human body is a seamless web of interconnecting systems, all of which contribute to its functional unity and healing capacity. Getting a handle on these vast, interconnected biological networks could lead to insights into a variety of diseases and greatly diminish or even eradicate them.

For the first time, *Quantum Medicine* presents information on a new class of natural antiviral/anti-infective compounds designed to augment the functioning of the immune system, including especially the liver, the body's primary cleansing organ.

The American Academy of Quantum Medicine educates and certifies doctors in Quantum Medicine to:

- Expand awareness and sensitivity for diagnosing the environmental stressors underlying illness;

- Boost the immune system and QEF in the rising number of immunocompromised and infected patients;

- Find effective ways to allow the immune system to defend itself against the mounting number of treatment-resistant germs and prevent *carcinogenesis,* that is, the earliest stages of cancer;

- Provide superior nourishment that is nontoxic, nonirradiated, and is not genetically modified, that can be absorbed and assimilated by the least healthy patients.

The new tools of Quantum Medicine probe and define the molecular and sub-molecular fabric of DNA instability and altered genetic expression, which give rise to pain, inflammatory disorders, and a long list of multi-system illnesses. These biotechnologies are stimulating doctors to ask new questions about the etiology of illness, the answers to which are providing a degree of power with which they may take control of mankind's greatest health enemies: infection and genetic or DNA instability.

WHAT YOU WILL FIND IN THIS BOOK

In this book, you'll discover powerful lifestyle changes you can make that will dramatically increase the flow of your healing energies. Like water flowing in a mountain stream with its dynamic, persevering, and yielding force, you'll feel the effortless and natural unfolding of your own vital healing energy as it awakens and interconnects with the entirety of your body's physiology. As you discover the potential you have to awaken your inner healer, you'll learn how to create optimal health. You'll enhance your intuition and your health in concert with these subtle rhythms of life.

You're about to embark on an educational journey that will teach you how to de-stress and enhance your body's innate wisdom and healing capacity. You'll benefit from the discoveries of this new field of Quantum Medicine by following the self-help guidelines in this book. Presented is the latest information that will help you:

- Harness the miraculous healing powers of your body's own quantum energy field (QEF);

- Learn how to eliminate harmful stressors that block or impede your ability to heal and repair damage;

- Boost your immune system so it can fight infections with more vigor and strength; and

- Stabilize your DNA to evoke the full power and unity of your QEF.

In the first two chapters, we will explore the origins of Quantum Medicine and the validation of its approaches. We will then examine the body itself, its healing powers, and the battles it must fight against invaders of all kinds, including stress. Next, we'll look at the healing foods, our allies in the fight against disease, and at the brain, our most powerful organ. We will make valuable recommendations regarding Quantum Foods incorporated into the Quantum Energy Diet. We'll even provide mouth-watering recipes that will make healthy eating both nutritious and delightful! You will find the Appendix and Resource section useful for eliminating toxins and poisons from your household, for contacting professional health practitioners, and for further reading.

In writing this book, I have always kept you, the reader, in mind. I want nothing less than your health and happiness. But you have to be a partner with me. You have to take the recommendations seriously and take part in your own improved health regimen. This probably means you must change—change the way you shop, the way you eat, the way you exercise, and even the way you think. But I am convinced it will be worth it, because it will be a vast change for the better! As your body's healing ability doubles, triples, and expands its boundaries to make extraordinary health and wellness a reality in your life, you'll feel a vitality you have never felt before. There will be a new you, and you will be better in every way possible.

1

The Birth of Quantum Medicine

Millions of Americans are suffering with disorders that are not responsive to medical treatment. Many live their lives with endless pain. Others are incapacitated by and/or die needlessly from diseases for which there are no effective medical treatments. Chronic fatigue and dangerous obesity are the most common complaints of a generation that has lost touch with the body's inner healing dimension.

An estimated 40 million Americans suffer from allergic disorders. Many individuals are finding themselves hypersensitive or allergic to substances that didn't bother them in the past. Other individuals are complaining that their allergies are changing and becoming even worse. They complain of having a runny nose, itchy, watery eyes, sneezing, skin rashes, and breathing difficulties that tend to roller coaster with the seasons. Since each season brings its own characteristic triggers, avoiding allergic reactions is not easy, as in many instances allergens that are in the air and in the environment year-round may be impossible to avoid.

While individual genetics, age, environment, and overall poor health combine to create allergic reactions, increasing worldwide pollution coupled with overcrowding, contaminated water and food, and indoor air contaminants overload the immune system and intensify allergic symptoms. Escalating levels of pollutants often build up in the body exceeding and incapacitating the body's natural detoxification capabilities. When this happens, common indoor air contaminants from synthetic cleaning agents and synthetic colognes, perfumes, body-care products, and air fresheners further infiltrate and damage delicate immune pathways. Detoxification mechanisms fail as nutrient reserves needed by the liver to keep the lymphatic system and immune system healthy are depleted. In an attempt to guard the body against this toxic overload, the immune system stimulates the release of a number of inflammatory chemicals, including histamine. When we present our doctor with these complaints, he or she is trained to block these chemical reactions with pharmaceuticals. Thus, the underlying causes of our illness remain obscured and masked by antihistamines, decongestants, cortisone, and anti-inflammatory drugs.

Between 15 and 37 percent of the American population consider themselves sensitive or allergic to chemicals, car exhaust, tobacco smoke, air fresheners, and the scents of many common household cleaning agents and body-care products. Some allergic individuals have to contend with headaches, seizures, fainting, dizziness, extreme fatigue, muscle or joint pain, asthma, sinusitis, insomnia, irregular heartbeat, maldigestion, depression, and anxiety or panic attacks when they are exposed to a potential allergen.

Each year there is a greater prevalence of complex, multi-system disorders many of which doctors dismiss as psychosomatic.

Every year, influenza is responsible for the deaths of 20,000 people in the United States, and millions worldwide are infected with some virus that eventually contributes to their death. Emerging viral illness can overwhelm an immuno-compromised patient. In such persons, a virus can replicate at lightning speed and invade every cell of the body, causing a wide spectrum of life-threatening disorders.

Millions who suffer with treatment-resistant syndromes also experience elevated rates of anxiety, depression, and other debilitating mental conditions. In mainstream medicine, the cause-and-effect relation between the syndrome involved and the psychiatric disorder is widely debated because it is often difficult to determine which condition is antecedent and which is consequent. Nonetheless, the prevalence of mental symptoms is clearly greater in patients with treatment-resistant syndromes than in the general population, or in similar groups of medically ill patients. For example, the prevalence of psychiatric symptoms is significantly greater in patients with fibromyalgia or irritable bowel syndrome, in patients with multiple chemical sensitivity, and in patients with chronic fatigue syndrome, than, for example, in patients with rheumatoid arthritis, or in healthy persons.

The body's natural healing cycles are being disrupted by:

- **Acid Overload.** Too much acidity in the body is harmful. It causes a reduction in healing energy and a depletion of key minerals needed to stay healthy. In Chapter 5, you'll learn how to quickly maintain the right acid/alkaline balance, or pH;

- **Toxin Overload.** An inability of the body to effectively neutralize and elimi-nate environmental toxins. Coupled with harmful electromagnetic pollutants, toxic overload scrambles and disorganizes our quantum energy field (QEF) and hormonal messages;

- **DNA Instability.** Altered gene expression can sabotage fertility, weaken the immune system, accelerate aging, erode intelligence, and activate powerful inflammatory processes that lead to the onset of many high-profile diseases. Studies from every corner of the globe confirm that DNA instability is behind cancer and all degenerative disease and is the central force behind a reduc-tion in our QEFs;

- **Chronic Infections.** The Centers for Disease Control reported a 139 percent increase in incidence of infection in the past ten years.

QEF: THE BODY'S QUANTUM ENERGY FIELD

Quantum Medicine begins with the assumption that the best way to heal the body is to enlist its help and heed its counsel. Medicine is at its best when it works with the body. By expanding and exploiting the body's myriad resources and taking advantage of its finely tuned physiology, we can make ourselves stronger and healthier. In order to reach our full potential, however, we need to understand how the body keeps itself in equilibrium, and how it rebalances itself when equilibrium is disrupted.

Our bodies already come equipped with all the necessary biological com-ponents of healing. The secret is found in the body's multi-leveled communi-cation networks consisting of light energies (called *biophotons*), hormones, and electrochemical information, and in understanding why and how they mal-function.

Over the course of the last century, and especially in the most recent decades, scientists from varied disciplines, such as molecular biology, quantum physics, and medical physiology, have been working diligently to provide solid, scientific proof that the human body is controlled and regulated by a quantum energy field (QEF)—a network of innumerable biophotons, which acts like an extremely fast supercomputer in the body. Both Chinese and Ayurvedic medi-cines acknowledge a body system of meridians, through which flows an ener-getic and information-laden "substance." This somewhat elusive substance is known in Chinese medicine as *chi* or *qi,* while Ayurvedic medicine acknowledges it as *prana.*

The meridians themselves are made up of clusters of electrically polarized molecules, and while research has yet to absolutely confirm this, it is most likely that these clusters are composed of water molecules. These water clusters have "permanent dipole moment," which means that they have an excess of positive charges on one end and negative charges on the other end. In Chinese medical terms, the positive and negative charges are known as "yin" and "yang," and it is the balancing of these charges that connotes health and wellness, and promotes optimal flow of energy through the body's meridian system, or QEF.

A strong, coherent QEF makes us feel totally alive, alert, and resilient to environmental stressors, while a weak, chaotic QEF results in sluggishness, fatigue, and sickness. Weak QEFs may be compared to an electrical system with poorly insulated wires, or improperly connected circuits, which cause the system to short-circuit or malfunction.

While we may marvel at the ingenuity of current scientific research, many of these discoveries simply confirm what practitioners of Ayruveda and Chinese Medicine have been teaching for thousands of years: The QEF is the life force that *governs* and *regulates* all cycles of natural healing in the body.

BIOPHOTONS: THE NEGLECTED DIMENSION OF HEALING

All living organisms possess a quantum energy field (QEF) and correspondingly emit light radiations called *biophotons* that are crucial to how efficiently the body's supercomputer controls and regulates biological processes. Every human thought and action is accompanied by electrical activity in the nervous system and by biophoton communication among cells. Indeed, life would not exist without the flow of meridian energies. In healthy individuals, biophotons are highly organized, tiny packets of light energy that are strong and plentiful. In sick organisms, however, biophoton light emissions are weak and chaotic. The body's acupuncture system of meridians directs this light energy to specific areas of the body, reenergizing function and vitality. New discoveries concerning biophotons and the QEF are helping to provide scientific explanations for the following:

- **Cell renewal.** Cells renew themselves at the amazing speed of 7–10 million times per second. Long ago, scientists had concluded that the lightning-fast speed of cell renewal simply cannot be explained on a physical level;

- **The speed of chemical reactions.** More than 100,000 chemical reactions occur per second in every cell of the body;

- **The speed of biological transmission.** If the information transmitted by the body were printed, it would take 100 years to read;

- **The human genome.** Biophotons allow DNA to store *libraries* of information in a sub-microscopic package;

- **Homeopathic medicine.** How homeopathy works (and why it doesn't work in some cases);

- **Aging.** According to both ancient wisdom and new scientific data, invigorating and balancing the body's meridian system makes it possible for us to lengthen our lives and enhance our later years;

- **The innate intelligence of living things.** The *coherence* or high degree of order and intelligence in all living things allows the body to carry out multiple tasks at the same time.

Biophotons unlock the secrets of how we heal ourselves, and how fish, insects, and birds create perfect and instant coordination. For instance, while each insect in a colony seems to have its own task, which it performs mutely, the seamless integration of all activities is, in fact, occuring through biophoton signals, which, to the degree of their coherence, contribute to the cooperation and organization throughout the colony. Dubbed "swarm intelligence" by biologists, the application of this innate functional coherence as a model of the human healing system is part and parcel of Quantum Medicine.

Unfortunately, however, the implicit assumption of modern medicine is that cells are just collections of independent biochemical pathways. But this is far from the reality. We can't understand cells by taking them apart piece by piece, because they function within crisscrossing biochemical pathways, branching and merging with biophotons to form complex communications networks. It is only when the parts of the human anatomy are working together in harmony by means of the QEF that the body can and will find more efficient ways to heal itself and defend itself against disease.

Biophotons are the driving force behind life. For example, *molecular coherence*—the way simple molecules assemble into complex structures—is governed by a variety of frequencies. Biophotons act as master regulators of the body's functions, discharging different frequencies at specific times to "switch on" different biological processes and unify the entire body in accordance with the body's needs. (See Figure 1.1 on page 12.) However, just as signals to your cell phone can be blocked in a mountainous area, biophoton signals can be blocked or diminished by stressors in the body. As a result, the body fails to efficiently transmit, receive, decode, store, interpret, and answer biological signals throughout specific systems of the body, losing its capacity to unify and control its defense and healing mechanisms. When these mechanisms are balanced and coherent, the body is "well." Thus, biophoton incoherence represents a loss of stability, causing an alteration in the harmonious oscillation rates of cells, which then can spread throughout the whole system, leading to dysfunction and imbalances in the body.

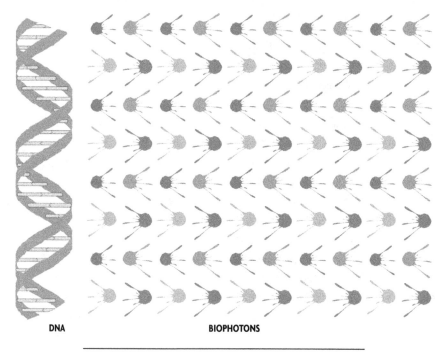

DNA   BIOPHOTONS

FIGURE 1.1. DNA and Coherent Biophoton Communication.

Given the complexity of biophoton signal transmission, one might expect that research in this discipline would be limited and too difficult to apply to healthcare problems. Nothing could be further from the truth. Research from the International Institute of Biophysics is showing that it is the body's QEF (not germs and genes) that determines whether we are healthy or ill.

Therefore, it is clear that the best way to treat disease and the aging process is to correct the disturbances or imbalances in the body's QEF. Assessing this highly informational system will give us clues as to what causative factors (stressors) underlie an individual's illness. These may be chemical toxins, nutritional deficiencies or imbalances, undetected pockets of infection, dental problems, electromagnetic pollution, allergens, or certain foods. Diagnosing these causes of an energy block or a disruption or distortion in the body's QEF can help to elicit powerful healing mechanisms.

THE CRITICAL NEED TO DEFINE STRESS IN OUR LIVES

Stress overload can wrench the emotions, impair organ function, diminish biological integrity, derange body chemistry, and literally extinguish life. Stress becomes a problem in our lives when it is chronic and when the impact outlasts or overwhelms the body's defenses and critically depletes our QEF. (Later in this book, you will learn how to thwart this process.) Mainstream medicine has accepted the fact that stress contributes to asthma, ulcers, ulcerative colitis, and other diseases. Yet because stress comes in many forms, there have been very few attempts to assess the underlying stress factors in a person's illness. Instead, drugs are used that mask the primary problem and ignore the wide spectrum of causative factors (stressors) that underlie human illness.

The most widely accepted theories about stress are based on the idea that emotions trigger biochemical or hormonal changes in the body. Nevertheless, none of these theories of modern psychiatry explains *how* environmental or lifestyle influences cause stress, or *why* they cause stress, or *how* these influences block the natural healing processes in the body.

My specific criticism of such ideas is that the "emotional" argument regarding stress flies in the face of the observable fact that stress ailments that initiate obvious measurable physical changes occur on a greater scale from environmental influences. Scientists attempt to measure such stress ailments in a variety of ways: using electrodermal biofeedback, measuring quantum meridian stress (QMSM), examining where body energy is too high or too low, noting where there may be a degenerative or inflammatory process at work, or, as the FDA would have it, simply noting where there is a physical indication of stress. In thousands of test-retest situations involving such calculations, we have observed that pent-up energies are suddenly released (like opening a clogged drain) when the appropriate remedy or supplement is given to a patient. Once released, these energies race down the meridian pathways into organs to stimulate the healing and repair mechanisms. The organs then absorb nourishment and detoxify themselves at faster, more efficient rates.

Accounting for the extraordinary prevalence of stress and how it causes blocks of the QEF requires that we find new ways of thinking about the nature of health and illness. The argument that emotions are the primary cause of illness can be ended abruptly as the patient who, after a QMSM, takes an appropriate nutrient and discovers that the emotions he or she had experienced for years were simply caused by lifestyle or environmental stressors. We have witnessed literally hundreds of depression and anxiety cases that were instantly cleared of these negative emotions when nutritional deficiencies or energetic blocks were corrected.

The impact of environmental stress is so prevalent in modern life that the chances of everyone incubating a stress disease are nearly 100 percent. Fibromylagia, chronic fatigue syndrome, leaky gut syndrome—all involve the excess storage of toxins in the joints and connective tissue, as well as a loss in the unity and power in the QEF to quickly heal and repair damage from these disorders.

However, since there is, as yet, insufficient understanding in mainstream medicine of how these unseen stressors affect the human body, most people who are ill are almost always *informationally deprived* as well. This lack of information creates additional stress, and the cycle of damage accelerates.

For example, studies in Quantum Medicine have shown that excruciating and frequent headaches most commonly involve a blockage or irritation in the gallbladder meridian. When patients simply eliminate the dietary stressors blocking gallbladder energies, headaches stop. Patients who constantly suppress headaches with painkillers never get to understand the underlying causes of their pain, so their headaches keep coming back. As a result, the obstruction of their gallbladder becomes an obstruction of their liver and nervous system, with severe and possibly life-threatening consequences.

Becoming aware that you need information also stirs up hopes that with the right kind of information, you'll get better. Fears about the unknown origins of an illness disappear, and with the right information, feelings of guilt dissipate. Once your wholeness and harmony are restored, your body will be less susceptible to assaults, whether chemical, infectious, or emotional. You'll have natural antidotes to compensate for the wounds and bruises inflicted by stress, and they will make you more resilient, more confident, and stronger.

Stress exacerbates and perpetuates physical and mental symptoms in treatment-resistant syndromes. For example, people who are obese often overeat in response to chemical toxins blocking their hormonal control systems, or such people may allow stress to deplete certain nutrients needed to metabolize fat.

In general, scientists recognize four major types of stress:

- **Lifestyle stresses** involving actions that throw our minds and bodies out of their natural balance (for example, excesses, such as overwork or overeating; deficiencies, such as drug or alcohol abuse; and psychological addictions);

- **Daily life stress** such as work deadlines or accidents that cause a loss of work time and thus a loss of income; adjusting to life changes, such as illness or being mentally or physically diminished in any way;

- **Major life stress** such as changes in employment, divorce, especially those involving custody battles, property settlements, mid-life crisis, death of a friend or loved one, a diagnosis of life-threatening or life-altering illness;

- **Environmental stress** involving weather (as in the case of seasonal affective disorder), pollutants, allergens, radiation, artificial light, viruses, bacteria, fungi, and high noise levels.

MY PERSONAL HEALTH JOURNEY: DISCOVERING QUANTUM MEDICINE

I began a journey that would eventually lead me to the development of the field of Quantum Medicine when I was fourteen years old. At that time, I was following the medical advice of physicians who had prescribed synthetic cortisone for my allergies and asthmatic condition. Over the next five years of treatment, there were danger signs: my hearing level dropped, and I suffered from chronic fatigue, migraine headaches, dizziness, and chronic kidney problems. Searching for answers to why I was getting sicker and going deaf, I consulted with medical specialists. I experienced endless frustration as doctor after doctor told me to "learn to live with" these disorders.

In 1973, at the age of nineteen, I underwent extensive medical testing at a world-renowned medical clinic. The tests revealed Allport's syndrome, a set of symptoms associated with a fatal kidney disease. I was told I would die within a year. At the same time, while my hearing loss was almost total, I was suffering from loud, annoying internal noises. I heard buzzing, roaring, ringing, and explosions! Without exaggerating, I can say that it was extremely difficult to maintain my sanity.

Despairing of receiving help from the doctors who had effectively presented me with a death sentence, I decided to take matters into my own hands. After consulting the *Physician's Desk Reference* (PDR), I began to suspect that my worsening health problems were due to side effects of the synthetic cortisone.

Realizing I had reached the limits of traditional medicine, I desperately worked to wean myself off that cortisone.

I immersed myself in a study of nutritional and herbal medicine. I realized that to save my own life, I would have to learn how to restore and maintain my body's lost healing abilities. My goal was to get my body to produce its own cortisone, naturally, to heal itself, in effect.

I made every effort to maintain fitness while experimenting with different diets and nutritional regimens. In this process, I discovered that the function of my cortisone-damaged kidneys began improving with the daily consumption of certain foods, as did my body's other healing processes. Later, through more experimentation with nutrition and dietary factors, I discovered different plant-based foods that further optimized my health. For example, I discovered that by altering the fat content and pH (acid or alkaline balance) of my diet, I could enhance detoxification and natural hormone production in my body.

In my quest for a diet and nutritional program that would save my life, I came across many nutritional teachings that turned out to be false, even detrimental to my health. For instance, when nutritional experts advised me to avoid fats, my blood cholesterol levels remained high, and I started gaining weight, feeling tired, and losing my mental clarity. It was as if someone had turned off the flow of my healing energies.

I began to look at fats and nutrition from a new perspective, as generators of healing energy and producers of hormones. I experimented with various nutritional factors, altering my diet to include, among other things, olive oil and raw coconut oil, sunflower seeds, almonds, and pumpkin seeds. Within only two weeks, my serum cholesterol was normalized! I felt energized and healthier than ever before. Life seemed rich and shimmering with possibilities, and I felt connected to something greater and vaster than I could ever have imagined. For the first time in my life, I felt creative, productive, and full of dynamic energy.

After much trial and error, I had discovered that it was specific combinations of plant-based nutrients that had made the difference. This newfound understanding stimulated my interest in the relationship between diet and healing and laid the foundational principles for what would become Quantum Medicine. Twenty-two years of subsequent exhaustive research and clinical experience have helped me to gain an understanding of how the body's healing mechanisms are nourished and organized with plant-based nutrients.

In association with another physician, I had the opportunity to see people with an array of clinical symptoms follow my dietary theories and return one or two months later, relieved of their symptoms. What these people experienced was not a placebo effect, but real results through feeding their bodies foods and nutrients that improved the power of their innate healing mechanisms.

Strengthening the relationship of our patients' QEF with their ailing physical bodies was our primary goal. We had discovered that reshaping faulty energy patterns through proper diet brought the whole body into greater harmony with itself, establishing well-being and, where needed, facilitating healing. Moreover, we discovered ways to target and heal specific organs and systems of the body.

I saw patients' long-term allergic symptoms end; fatigue vanish; blood pressure normalize; pain, headaches, anxiety, and inflammation disappear; hearing and vision improve; and various degenerative conditions improve dramatically despite years of unsuccessful medical management. These profound clinical successes were based on increasing the flow of the individual's healing energies through dietary changes while de-stressing their bodies, detoxifying them of harmful substances. That we got results quickly in patients who had been debilitated for years with seemingly treatment-resistant syndromes was proof that we'd tapped into the body's latent healing powers.

My research colleagues and I studied hundreds of plants and whole foods to find the natural medicines that would initiate healing through the reorganization and enhancement of the body's QEF. Our search was rewarded with the discovery of rare herbals that can revitalize and strengthen the connection between an individual's QEF and his or her body, resulting in a state of "quantum coherence." By such a state, we mean the highest level of order or organization within the human organism, according to the International Institute of Biophysics, which is composed of fifteen groups of scientists from university centers around the world. According to their research, healthy individuals have exquisite coherence at the quantum level, while sick individuals with weak immune systems or cancer have chaotic or very poor coherence, with disturbed biophoton cellular communications. The process of revitalizing disrupted QEFs was further enhanced when we blended these healing herbs in specific proportions. Our discoveries of superior health-promoting and energy-enhancing foods resulted in our developing a new class of medicinal food complexes, *quantum foods,* that would literally make one healthier with each bite one took.

Eventually, I blended Oriental medicine, Ayurveda, homeopathy, European and Native American herbology, naturopathy, nutrition and biochemistry, applied kinesiology/chiropractic, and therapeutic bodywork into my practice.

The combination of these healing modalities resulted in a clinical protocol that was far more potent and thorough than any one of them taken alone. By 1994, I called this blend of unique discoveries and ancient healing systems *Quantum Medicine*. Patients were typically telling me, "I've made more progress in just a few months than I've made in years with any other treatments."

THE ACCEPTANCE OF QUANTUM PRINCIPLES

According to a recent article in the *Scientific American*, "30 percent of the U.S. gross national product is based on inventions made possible by quantum mechanics, from semiconductors in computer chips to lasers in compact disc players, magnetic resonance imaging in hospitals, and much more."

Every human thought and action is accompanied by electrical activity in the nervous system and by biophoton communication among cells. Indeed, life would not exist without the flow of ions across the membranes of cells, and the ebb and flow of meridian energies.

As medicine more and more adopts the principles of quantum physics that are making such waves in other walks of life, current outdated symptom-based protocols will fade into the background. Already the principles of quantum physics have been behind a host of technological breakthroughs such as the development of MRI scanners and surgical lasers commonly used by physicians and dentists worldwide.

Before long, doctors will learn to tap into the body's supercomputer, the QEF. This window into the body's biological communication network will provide us with information about the hidden promoters and inducers of illness that jam our bodies' delicate healing and repair mechanisms so we can't get well. By acknowledging the body's innate intelligence, we will be able to selectively "turn off" faulty genetic patterns that give rise to many high-profile illnesses, such as Alzheimer's disease, Parkinson's disease, and fibromyalgia.

THE NEED FOR QUANTUM NOURISHMENT

Nobel Prize laureate Albert Szent-Györgyi has stated, "We live by a small trickle of electricity from the sun." The miracle of photosynthesis transforms the sun's light energies into green plants, trees, grasses, and medicinal herbs. True nourishment must accomplish two tasks:

1. It must allow assimilation of the full spectrum of this light energy throughout the body to compensate for QEF losses caused by environmental and life stress, and

2. It must couple this light energy with living nutrients that are rapidly absorbed and assimilated into the cells of our bodies.

Unfortunately, the overwhelming majority of natural supplements provided by today's nutritionists and dieticians do not fill this bill. Instead, more than 97 percent of today's nutritional supplements are void of light energy and contain mostly synthetic (man-made) nutrition as well as stress-inducing toxins, instead of living food nourishment! These supplements stimulate chemical energy and deplete quantum energy. Here's the real danger: When we stimulate our bodies through *improper* foods, supplements, and drugs, we deplete nutrients and electrons needed to protect us from the chaotic and unhealthy conditions of our modern world, and we suppress our QEF. An example of this would be eating processed white sugar as opposed to obtaining sugar in a natural form, such as from fruit or honey. The fruit or honey would contain additional nutrients, by which the body can metabolize the sugar content. But the processed sugar lacks these additional nutrients, so the body must "borrow" those nutrients from its own storage sites. Thus, while the sugar may seem like a stimulant, an energizer, it actually is depleting our energy stores.

Quantum nourishment (which will be discussed in Chapter 10) helps to organize and energize the body's QEF. Each of our cells vibrates with energy because of crystal-like structures that resonate to different light energies or frequencies of biophotons. Quantum nutrients are propelled deeply into each cell where they quickly energize the cell's functions with healthy resonant frequencies, enhancing the bioavailability of nutrients, accelerating enzyme functions, and driving the regenerative functions in the body (see Figure 1.2 on page 20).

Meridian energy flow, when assessed through QMSM biofeedback systems, documents how different plants with varying frequencies can organize and balance the body. Atoms and molecules are excited by the energies of specific resonances, thereby creating a primary force to help us regain or sustain our health. Here are some common examples of the principle of resonance:

- The singer who hits a note that is the precise resonant frequency of a wine glass is able to shatter the glass;

- Plucking the E string of a violin will cause another violin on the opposite side of a room to vibrate without being touched. The E strings of the violins are like the electrons and atoms, which react only if they are exposed to energy of their resonant frequency;

- Homeopathy, used by thousands of doctors worldwide, works on the principle of resonance. A particular remedy is able to reproduce the symptoms of a sick person in a healthy individual. Similarly, a correctly chosen homeopathic remedy's frequency pattern will resonate with the frequency of a patient's illness, allowing the body's energetic system to assimilate the needed energy, thereby regulating the body toward health.

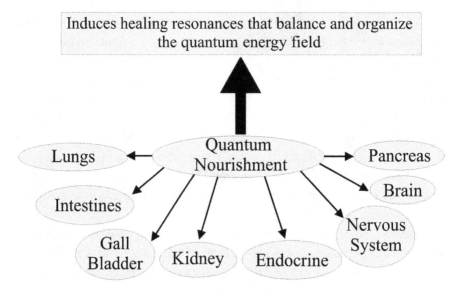

FIGURE 1.2. Quantum nourishment provides physical and energetic nourishment to balance the quantum energy field.

Through quantum nourishment, we can establish a link between the physical and the energetic bodies, and combat the discord of negative lifestyles that overstimulate the body. Quantum nourishment promotes superior coherence and stability in DNA patterns so our cells can divide properly and our organs function and heal efficiently.

When 1999 Nobel Prize winner Dr. Gunter Blobel stated, "Each protein carries in its structure the information needed to specify its proper location in the cell," he presaged the development of the principle of quantum nourishment, that is, using high-quality proteins of resonant frequencies to carry physical nourishment to the cells, allowing healing and regeneration to take place.

An optimum food, therefore, is one that will transfer, in an organized way, healing and rejuvenation energies into our biological systems. In more than thirty years of research, I have identified certain foods that provide true quantum nourishment, above and beyond other ordinary foods and vitamins. Furthermore, as the research of the American Academy of Quantum Medicine scientists confirms, there is a 10- to 100-fold increase in the transfer of energetic patterns into our QEF when these foods are properly grown, harvested, prepared, and combined in specific proportions.

STRENGTHENING AND EXPANDING THE BODY'S QEF

Quantum Medicine recognizes the importance of the whole person in dealing with health and illness, as the QEF sustains all physiological functioning. Neglect of this entity causes the quality of life to become diminished. Energy shortages slow down the body's immune defenses against viruses and microbes. But with the information in this book, you'll learn how to realign your healing energies in a precise, orderly arrangement. You'll learn that premature aging, physical degeneration, and clusters of symptoms that never seem to go away can now be reversed and/or eliminated.

If you follow the guidelines in this book, you will be able to achieve the relief of stubborn symptoms and long-term health problems, as I did. This is the first and most important benefit of strengthening and expanding your body's QEF. However, you will also notice an overall enhancement of your ability to detect subtle stressors, to perceive the world and its patterns of ever-increasing levels of complexity with greater ease and precision. Perhaps for the first time in a long time, you will be a whole person.

The Scientific Validation of Quantum Medicine

In 1918, Max Planck, one of the greatest physicists of all time, was awarded a Nobel Prize for his research that led to the development of quantum physics. A basic tenet of quantum physics is that absolutely everything has a frequency. Each cell of our bodies has its own ideal frequency. When this frequency is al tered through various stress factors, so is the communicating capability of our biophotons (see Figure 2.1), and sickness is often the result. Planck's breakthrough research provided the foundational principles that today underlie Quantum Medicine.

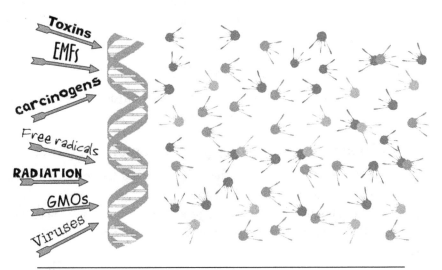

FIGURE 2.1. DNA-induced Stress Causing Chaotic Biophoton Communication.

Quantum Medicine is a combination of many different health-assessment protocols, resulting in a single, energy-based medical paradigm. These protocols increase the likelihood of jump-starting weak or disordered healing mechanisms in diseased people, and raise hopes that someday soon quantum therapies will heal numerous degenerative diseases, including Parkinson's disease, Alzheimer's disease, and multiple sclerosis, as well as providing a powerful arsenal of weapons against stroke, heart trauma, and cancer. Quantum Medicine views disease as a disruption or distortion of the body's QEF. Rather than suppressing the symptoms (such as pain and inflammation) of this disharmony, Quantum Medicine approaches illness with the intent of eliminating the disharmony, either with bursts of energy or with stimulations of a specific resonance that correct the disharmony and promote innate healing.

Moreover, the quantum medical model holds the promise of extending our life spans and overall well-being by *preventing* stroke, heart disease, diabetes, and other degenerative diseases.

More and more today, we are hearing the words of Hippocrates echoed: "Our natures are physicians of our diseases." The true message of optimal health, then, is that we need to direct our attention to the wisdom of the body, listen to it carefully, and respond once we are aware of conflicts. If we are to have any hope of understanding the body, and of exploring its true potential for healing, we first need a clear understanding of what "healing" really is; what is myth and what is useful theory; what has been ignored or neglected by modern medicine; and above all, where the extraordinary dimensions of healing are located in the body.

QUANTUM MEDICINE: THE BEGINNINGS

There are two approaches to Quantum Medicine: Western and Eastern. Because they are so different in conception, I will discuss each separately.

Western Foundational Beginnings of Quantum Medicine

As I've indicated at the beginning of this chapter, it was the research of Max Planck that led to his own discovery of quantum physics and the realization that everything emits a frequency. Since then, a panoply of related research has built upon his findings and laid a solid foundation for the guiding principles of Quantum Medicine.

It was the research of Dr. Harold Saxton Burr at Yale University in the 1920s and 1930s that extended Planck's quantum discoveries to different forms of life. Burr researched the energetic qualities of different flora and fauna, noticing changes in the electrical fields of trees, for example, that correlated to seasonal changes, sunlight and darkness, cycles of the moon, and sunspots. In humans, he noted that emotional stress affected the body's energy field. Observing hormonal changes in women, he was able to record an increased voltage just before ovulation and a subsequent drop in voltage just as the egg was released. Moreover, Burr and his colleagues were able to identify malignant tissues and predict when a woman would develop cancer of the cervix—all based on observing and monitoring voltage changes in her body. Burr summarized his forty-three years of research in his book *Blueprint for Immortality: The Electric Patterns of Life.* This breakthrough research revealed important scientific discoveries:

1. All living things, from humans to mice, from trees to seeds, are formed and controlled by QEFs, which Burr called *L fields;*

2. L fields are the basic blueprints of all life;

3. L fields are informational and can be used to diagnose physical and mental conditions before the symptoms of an illness develop.

A brief overview of the events of the following years will help us to put the Western approach in context and understand the development of the concepts that support Quantum Medicine:

• An American neurologist, Albert Abrams, M.D., who taught pathology at Stanford University's medical school during the early 1900s, observed that since pathological tissue emitted atypical resonances or waves, these waves could be used with great accuracy to locate and treat an infection or pathology. In one experiment, resonant frequencies or radiations from quinine eliminated the resonances associated with malaria, and in another, mercurial salts stopped syphilis radiations. Other experiments with other known antidotes produced similar results;

• In a series of twenty-five clinical trials performed during the 1920s, Dr. William Boyd confirmed Abrams's research. With 100 percent accuracy, he was able to identify chemicals and tissues within the human body without visual or any other clues except their resonances. In 1924, the Royal Society of Medicine investigated Boyd's claims and found them valid;

• Another researcher, George Lakhovsky, published *The Secret of Life* in 1925, in which he observed that "every living cell is essentially dependent on its nucleus, which is the center of oscillations and gives off radiations."

Lakhovsky defines vitality and disease as a battle between the healthy resonances of cells and the unhealthy, alien resonances of microbes and other
toxins.

Using the sun as an analogy, we can grasp the importance of Lakhovsky's
observation to the field of Quantum Medicine. The sun is the center of our
solar system, and life could not exist without the sun giving off radiations
that set up oscillations in living matter. In like manner, atoms are the center of
our biological systems, and without the energy radiations emanating from our
cells, our lives could not survive. The same energy principles, in other words,
that work on the macroscopic level in the world around us work on the
microscopic level in the world within us;

- Famous U.S. surgeon and founder of the Cleveland Clinic in Ohio, George
  Crile, M.D., supported Lakhovsky's finding with independent studies that were
  reported in his book *The Phenomena of Life: A Radio-Electric Interpretation,*
  published in 1936. "Electricity is the energy that drives the organism," he said.
  He likened the cell to a battery and stated, "It is clear that in the second half
  of life the electrical potential of the elderly patient as a whole or of this or
  that organ, has been very much reduced and that by so much, the margin of
  safety [vis-a-vis good health and vitality] has been dangerously diminished";

- In the *British Medical Journal* in 1937, Sir Thomas Lewis described an independent cutaneous nerve system of pathways that was not composed of
  nerve fibers, but was rather electromagnetic;

- Further documentation of the body's electromagnetic energies came from
  photographic techniques, the discovery of which, in Russian, in 1949, is generally credited to Semyon Kirlian. With the interaction of a high-frequency
  electric discharge and a photographic plate, he captured the energetic im-
  prints of living organisms on film. Further research performed during the
  1950s by scientists at the Kirov State University of Kazakhstan, and by M. K.
  Gaikin, M.D., correlated these measurements with traditional Chinese medicine concepts of energy flow;

  Some of the most impressive work with Kirlian photography appears in
  Peter Mandel's 1988 book *Energy Emission Analysis.* Mandel's discovery, based
  on more than 800,000 energy emission analysis (EEA) photographs, documented the beginning and end points of classical acupuncture. Numerous
  irregularities of bodily functions were clearly observable in the photographs,

and Mandel based his therapeutic intervention on either the positive or negative EEA photographs;

- In 1977, using electromyography (EMG), that is, a measurement of the brain's
  electomagnetic activity, Dr. Valerie Hunt at the University of California, Los
  Angeles, discovered that the body emits oscillations that are measurable.
  With sophisticated equipment, Hunt was able to accurately monitor fluctua-
  tions in the body's electromagnetic energy levels;

- Dr. John Zimmerman of the University of Colorado School of Medicine used
  an ultra-sensitive magnetic field detector called a *Super-conducting Quantum Interference Device* (SQUID) to measure human energy fields. He found
  that the mere contact of human energy to enzymes causes a change in
  enzyme activity that mirrors natural cellular intelligence. Subtle energetic
  phenomena was also scientifically detected and measured by Dr. Valerie
  Hunt;

- Carlo Rubbia made an astounding observation on the importance of biological information fields, which, he reported, are far greater than the biochemical or molecular information in the human body. This observation was
  astounding because what it means is that examining only the physical body is
  assessing only a small part of the human organism. For this work, Rubbia
  received the Nobel Prize for Biology in 1984;

- A controlled research study on rats by the U.S. Naval Research Center, Bethesda, Maryland, published in *Biomagnetics* in 1986, documented that the magnetic resonance from lithium (administered homeopathically via injection
  rather than an oral dose) was able to subdue behavior and depress the central
  nervous system. This study is important because it documents significant biological effects from minute radiations that support the way homeopathic
  medicines work, namely, solely on the principle of resonant frequencies in a
  liquid with no chemical molecules;

- In his 1990 book, *Crosscurrents: The Perils of Electropollution,* Nobel Prize
  double-nominee, Robert O. Becker, M.D., reported that the electromagnetic
  resonance in the human body behaves in a similar fashion to magnetic resonance imaging (MRI), a noninvasive diagnostic technique used to produce
  images of atomic and molecular structures (especially of human cells, tissues,
  and organs), and that the body's innate resonances could be used to explain
  and heal problematic health issues.

Now that we have some understanding of the Western approaches to Quantum Medicine, let us examine the Eastern.

Eastern Foundational Beginnings of Quantum Medicine

Along with the impressive accumulation of proof for the QEF of the human body and the reliability of the QEF in revealing our true state of health, there has long been an Eastern healing modality based on restoring balance in the body's energy system. It is acupuncture, the true forerunner of Quantum Medicine. Yet in spite of thousands of years of proven efficacy, there still are many who remain skeptical of the authenticity of this ancient Chinese healing art.

Long before Western medicine and the pharmaceutical industry's development of the prevailing system of healing, ancient systems existed that recognized a balanced quantum energy system as the elixir of good health. According to Chinese medical experts, energy channels, called meridians, run through the entire human body. These meridians are responsible for the functioning of cells and the activation of the body's natural healing mechanisms. They themselves are activated and harmonized by *chi,* or vital energy, flowing through them. For thousands of years, one of the core tenets of traditional Chinese medicine has been the recognition of the role played by chi in sickness and disease. When our chi is strong and balanced, flowing smoothly through our meridians, we are healthy. When our chi is weak or becomes blocked, it can cause bodily imbalances and we become ill.

The following is a brief overview of the research that has been done to support the existence of acupuncture meridians:

- From 1960 to 1980, Reinhold Voll, M.D., who discovered electroacupuncture techniques, spent two decades studying acupuncture points and their related meridians. Voll discovered that almost all Chinese acupuncture points could be detected by a change in skin resistance (that is, a change in electrical voltage measured on the skin);

- During the 1960s, researchers injected the acupoints of animals with radioactive P (an isotope of phosphorus), measuring the uptake of the substance into surrounding tissues. When microautoradiography techniques were used to trace the injected substances, they discovered that the P followed the exact path of the classical acupuncture meridians;

- Studies done by Dr. Justa Smith in 1972 reveal that meridian energy can accelerate the kinetic activity of enzymes;

- In 1978, Dr. Hiroshi Motoyama's AMI Machine (short for apparatus for mea-suring the functions of the meridians and corresponding internal organ) assessed data on more than 5,000 patients, documenting strong correlations between weaker meridians and underlying disease states in associated organ systems;

- In 1985, Pierre de Vernejoul at the University of Paris injected radioactive markers in acupuncture points of human subjects. Using gamma-camera imaging, he tracked the movement of the isotope. His findings indicated that the tracer followed the pathways of the classical meridian lines at the speed of 30 centimeters in four to six minutes. As a control, he also made random injections in the skin, vessels, and lymphatic channels, documenting that there was no migration at these sites;

- In 1986, using electronographic body scans, researchers documented meridi-an pathways, and in studies similar to those undertaken by Dr. Burr in the 1920s and 1930s, Professor Kim found that the meridian ducts were formed within fifteen hours of conception in the embryonic chick, before even the rudimentary organs were formed;

- In another experiment, Professor Kim severed the liver meridian in a frog and observed the subsequent changes in the liver tissue. Shortly after severing the meridian, he discovered enlarged liver cells. Three days later, he noted serious vascular degeneration throughout the entire liver;

- In 1988, Dr. William A. Tiller of Stanford University observed close to a twenty-fold drop in electrical resistance at the exact center of the acupressure points.

Yet in spite of this impressive body of research on the underlying principles of Eastern medicine, for the most part, the scientific-political-social consensus on acceptable medical practices declines to acknowledge the idea of a self-governing healing entity in the body.

CURRENT STATUS

It would seem that all this credible research has been ignored by modern medi-cine. Why should that be so? My best guess is that medical scientists are torn between logical, substantive ideas and data about the potency of healing, and their practical need to conform to the convictions of their scientific peers, who disavow the idea that healing can be evoked naturally without drug intervention. In addition, they find it hard to accept scientific proof that is not published in their own medical journals, even though there is, in fact, in the vast archives of the sciences of physics and biology, a host of scientific reports that give exciting testimony to the extraordinary ranges of healing powers within each and every one of us. Because I've chosen, in this book, to report only what has been scientifically verified according to generally accepted research protocols, a great deal of the existing evidence has not been included. Nevertheless, it is obvious from the data presented that both evidence and logic lead to a conclusion that the body has a unique power to guide and control inner healing.

Traditional Chinese theories were developed thousands of years ago when the planet was not as polluted and food was not genetically engineered or depleted in nutrients. Today, the ancient healing art of acupuncture is no longer sufficient by itself. Old and outdated techniques have had to be revised and updated, according to the latest research, as well as fine-tuned to meet the challenges of the environment we live in today and are likely to encounter in the future. Quantum Medicine uses the meridian system as a way to determine organ responses to specific stressors, through a process called Quantum Meridian Stress Measurement (QMSM), described in the previous chapter.

In addition, advanced methods of thermographic analysis (using body temperature to detect inflammation, infection, and energetic and/or nerve blockages) have been improvised and used in Quantum Medicine research to assess and locate hidden blockages of energy flow, such as an infected root canal, scar tissue at an old surgical site, or functional and structural problems related to inefficiency in how the brain regulates the body through the oval cavity and teeth, technically referred to as *faulty brain proprioception.*

Your personal tools for self-healing have roots on the foundational principles described in this chapter. Each of chapters that follow will empower you to learn, practice, and share superior, clinically tested, ways of getting and staying well.

The Body's Incredible Innate Healing Powers

The healing energies that flow throughout living organisms, including the human body, are prodigious, awe-inspiring, and miraculous. When a salamander's leg is torn off by a predator, for example, the salamander simply regrows a new one. When a pond worm is chopped in half, each half regrows into a complete worm. How do these animals' bodies know how and where to reassemble new organs? The miraculous intelligence and power of regrowth are inherent in their QEFs. Why does this not seem to work also with the human body? Where have we gone wrong?

In humans, the genetic cascades of biophoton energies are the most powerful when we are embryos. The force and magnitude of this flow determines the course of our health. As we grow older and enter the world, our immune systems immediately engage in warfare against pathogens, chemicals, and other stressors. For reasons not yet fully understood, overengaging our immune systems has the effect of repressing healing networks within our DNA. While the event of any such thing happening is probably a long way off, plausible evidence exists to support the idea that by identifying and eliminating these stressors, we humans may be capable of feats of regeneration similar to those found in species like the salamander or pond worm.

Our capability for inner healing is so great that to explore the endless boundaries of its power would render helpless even the best of minds. The shortcoming of most current scientific study of the human body is that it only delves deeply into the chemistry and molecular nature of cells, giving very little attention to how healing functions can be nourished, expanded, or used more efficiently.

Biochemistry alone cannot explain life. Leading biochemists have documented that chemical reactions take place billions of times faster in the living body than in a test tube. This one fact should be sufficient to spur recognition of the critical importance of our QEF, its biophotonic activity—what we could rightly call the *life principle.*

Biochemists have encountered innumerable failures when they've tried to synthesize the building blocks of life or create life in a test tube. Without taking the life principle into consideration, they are doomed to even more failures.

Both buffeted and compelled by the rewards of political, medical, and pharmaceutical industry economics, most researchers have not probed the natural healing dimension of the body. This has been an unfortunate deterrent to understanding how to nurture, strengthen, and fulfill the body's healing abilities. But while researchers and mainstream doctors have their heads buried in the sand, ordinary people everywhere have begun to look inward to discover the long-hidden powers of the body. There is an ever-widening interest in alternative medicine and natural healing methods. Quantum Medicine makes a solid case for the existence of a superior intelligence with unimagined potency and range of healing powers within every person. From the sum of the evidence, I believe, emerges a human superpotential for innate healing.

HEALING POWERS AND LIGHT ENERGIES

Healing power is all around us in the form of sunlight, which emits biopohton energy, vital to all life on earth. New biotechnologies that enable scientists to observe different frequencies of light energies in the universe have revealed that various galaxies in the universe emit photons of differing frequencies. Scientists have also discovered that photons drive chemical reactions that synthesize complex molecules, some of which are the building blocks of life as we know it.

Without full spectrum sunlight, some people suffer from seasonal affective disorder (SAD), a depression that deepens during the winter months when the hours of sunlight each day are shorter. Nowhere is the life-sustaining power of sun more evident than in the earth's polar regions where the risks for bone disease, rickets, and tooth decay run high unless people receive a daily dose of ultraviolet light.

It is biophotons (biological light energies) that regulate the body's QEF, which in turn, regulates the physical body. When a disruption or imbalance occurs in the body, health can be restored by therapies that *nurture* and *activate* our light energy, which in turn does the following:

• stabilizes DNA and biophoton light energies;

- stabilizes and maintains pH;

- stabilizes and maintains detoxification functions of the body;

- stabilizes and enhances immune, brain, and hormonal functions.

Scientists in the chemical and molecular fields of medicine recognize that the cell can achieve extraordinary feats that cannot be explained in terms of existing chemical and medical models. In studying the intricate complexities of human functioning, scientific research often generates more questions than answers. Today, some of the most important questions in science and medicine are:

1. How can two meters of DNA—the nucleic acid in the nuclei of cells that directs all the activities of the cell—be packed into a space only one-hundredth of a millimeter across?

2. What is the driving force that directs the activity of trillions of cells into diverse and yet coherent functions?

3. What is the true source of intuitive healing?

INTUITION AND HEALING

Animals instinctively know how to nurse their young, what to eat when they're sick, or how to tend to other types of injuries. A similar intuitive wisdom is present also in the human body, though, for the most part, we tend to be unaware of it. Suppressed by overstimulation and excessive stress, the human body's intuitive powers have become diminished.

Our own human instinct, what we think of as intuition, is actually a function of our QEF. When energy flow runs unimpeded through our higher brain centers, we experience high levels of intuitive insight. Just as animals do, we sense and feel when something is not working properly in our bodies, when, for instance, a given organ is deficient or not functioning at an optimal level. And we also know by how we feel what we should eat in order to bring ourselves back to optimal health. We learn by sensing the immediate lifts or drops in energy after eating certain foods, even when these alterations are quite subtle.

Today, the ability to intuit the body's needs has been, for the most part, lost. Overloads of stressors, aided by our learned responses to them, have disrupted our delicate feedback systems and weakened our energetic-organ connections.

When we experience a symptom, we react with a learned response to the symptom, rather than a *felt* response to the *cause* of the symptom. Additionally, most of us eat by habit, that is, without listening to our bodies, so we are most often taking in foods that don't serve our overall well-being. We are oblivious to the signals our bodies are sending us through rises and falls in our energy levels. However, by eliminating stressor foods from our diet and consuming healing quantum foods that balance pH and raise energy levels, we can enhance our intuition, gaining access to a unique and powerful healing tool.

NEW RESEARCH ON BIOPHOTONS

Biophotonic and electromagnetic oscillations, which are present in the QEF of the living body, imbue life with its power and versatility. New research on biophotons has yielded some amazing conclusions, surprising even to physicists. For instance, studies have confirmed that biophotons do the following:

- transform the activities of millions of brain cells into coherent thoughts;

- contribute to the amazing teamwork and unity between the activities of millions of cells in the body;

- explain how DNA can hold such a vast amount of information in such a small space;

- explain how endless supplies of living tissue, grown from a single cell, can repair damage anywhere in the body; and

- explain, on the other hand, that if the information transmitted by the biophotons is incomplete, the same single cell could spread cancer anywhere in the body.

Understanding how frequency oscillations affect rates of biochemical reactions will have incredible consequences in the healthcare field. Imagine being able to subtly fine-tune the oscillations of diseased cells toward healthful oscillations, or being able to find answers to the uncontrolled cell death that takes place in disorders like Parkinson's disease and Alzheimer's disease. With electromagnetic assessment of total body regulation, it becomes possible to understand why sick cells fail to produce important compounds needed by the body to fight disease. Moreover, the difference between an active and inactive enzyme molecule, viewed as a subtle difference in electromagnetic frequency, may provide clues to many mysterious molecular processes underlying genetic mutations.

Quantum Medicine presumes that when we reverse abnormal energy, we create health. It sounds so simple, doesn't it? However, before we can reverse that negative energy, we need to understand the patterns generated by a wide spectrum of stress factors that give rise to disturbed cellular interactions and lead to malfunctions in the body.

MEDICAL TECHNOLOGY THAT ACKNOWLEDGES THE QEF

There are myriad electrical forces at work within the body—fundamental regulatory processes that involve many different kinds of electronic energy. Various instruments assess the body's electrical phenomena, including the following:

- **Electrocardiograph.** Measures the electrical activities from different areas of the heart;

- **Heart variability assessment.** Measures autonomic nervous balance in the heart itself;

- **Electroencephalograph.** Measures electrical activities from different areas of the brain;

- **Stress electrocardiogram.** Measures subtle changes in heart function in response to exercise;

- **Nystagmometry.** Records electrical information on eye movement after stimulating the inner ear with cold or hot water;

- **Galvanic skin response.** Measures electrical conductance between two electrodes placed on the skin while the patient is exposed to various stimuli;

- **Chinese gastrointestinal analysis.** Measures electrical activity of various areas of the gastrointestinal tract to diagnose ulcers, stomach cancers, colon disorders, and other digestive system abnormalities; while this is not a common practice of Western medicine, it is mainstream in Asia;

- **Electromyelography.** Measures electrical activity of muscles after nerve stimulation to predict the functional status of a specific muscle;

- **Brain stem audiometry:** Measures brain-wave activity in response to sounds;

- **Cochlear microphonics.** Measures electrical changes in the inner-ear function of the cochlea after sound-wave stimulation;

- **Magnetic resonance imaging (MRI).** measures magnetic resonant information to construct images of different structures of the body;

- **Electroacupuncture according to voll (EAV).** To gain useful diagnostic information about the meridian-organ connections of the body, EAV measures the precise level of current conducted to the acupuncture points after a low-voltage electrical charge has been introduced.

Again, for the person under stress, information is paramount to engaging healing energies to augment repair and regeneration. In essence, a doctor isn't a healer, but a facilitator who can guide your own body to accomplish the miracle of healing. Healing is an innate process already hardwired in all of us.

When we identify and decrease the stressors that derail or block healing, the body's healing energies once more are able to direct streams of light energy without interference. In the following chapters, we'll explore some of the factors that stress the body's natural healing mechanisms. You'll learn that in order to perform the complex functions of healing, the body must analyze, evaluate, and judge what is wrong. It might communicate its *dis-ease* in symptoms that you experience. When confronted with symptoms, it's important that we not suppress them. Rather, we should try to understand them. When our bodies' interpretive powers are hindered by stress overload (cluttered with daily doses of unwanted toxins, deficiencies and excesses, or interferences from electromagnetic pollution), it may be operating chaotically, without unity between its functional parts. Study after study has shown that these stressors can be eliminated or decreased enough to free the endless bounds of your QEF.

4

DNA and Oxidative Stress: Healing, Aging, and Cancer

The seemingly endless twine of the DNA double helix contains 60,000 to 100,000 genes encoded by 3 billion chemical parts. It is this intelligence that governs and regulates our growth from a single-fertilized egg to a fully developed human. It is this intelligence that keeps us alive, by regenerating our tissues, producing thousands of hormones and proteins necessary for our bodies to thrive, and revving up our immune systems when our bodies enter into combat with a lethal virus.

Our DNA, in other words, is the determining factor of what makes us human. Moreover, as a biophoton generator, DNA holds the key to life itself. DNA is the software on which we run. It is the life principle, and as such, it is paramount to our health destiny.

FREE RADICALS, OXIDATION, AND DNA DAMAGE

Life is dependent upon processing and communicating complex information at lightning-fast speeds. How effectively our DNA software runs depends upon its effective internal communication (as shown in Figure 1.1 on page 12) and its external communication with all facets of our anatomy.

Chemical pollutants in our air, water, and food initiate the release of unstable and, therefore, toxic oxygen molecules, known as "free radicals," in our bodies, causing cells to oxidize and become themselves electrically unstable. Free radicals are produced in limited amounts as a natural byproduct of our metabolism. But excess free radicals are caused by such stressors as cigarette smoke, X-rays, air pollutants, and food additives. Uninhibited, they are capable of destroying cells and glands that produce hormones. What we know as "chemical carcinogens" are really any chemical substances that, after transformation by normal human metabolic enzymes, become electron-*deficient* molecules. As such, they react readily with electron-*rich* molecules such as protein and DNA, which they latch on to in an effort to stabilize themselves.

The mitochondria is the cell's energy factory; it is important for cell metabolism because it converts food into usable cellular energy. As the mitochondria is also the site in the cell where the majority of oxidative chemistry occurs, mitochondrial DNA is some 2,000 times more susceptible to oxidative damage than nuclear DNA.

In his book *Our Stolen Future,* Theo Colborn points out that many of today's synthetic chemicals, because they are hormonally active compounds, wreak havoc in our bodies by scrambling healthy hormonal messages and altering gene expression to induce free radicals. In fact, these toxic compounds are light scramblers. They create chaos within biophoton transmissions, altering frequencies, degrading our QEF, and destabilizing DNA. With DNA instability, we erode intelligence, sabotage fertility, weaken the immune system, accelerate aging, and activate powerful inflammatory processes that lead to the onset of many high-profile diseases. Additionally, any time stress creates an Alarm Reaction in the body, we release free radicals.

Just as oxidation causes iron to rust, free-radical oxidation at the cellular level sets off a series of volatile chain reactions, damaging chemical compounds, DNA, hormone receptors, and other delicate cellular machinery. Free-radical oxidation also causes great harm to cells, tissues, and organs of the body. These reactions are called "oxidative stress," a condition that produces powerful chemicals that contribute to pain, inflammation in the body, aging, and carcinogenesis.

The body's antioxidant (free-radical fighters) defense system, consisting of enzymes, vitamins, phytochemicals, and other nutrients, neutralizes these free radicals. It also protects its own cells by employing special enzymes that serve as quencher molecules to break free-radical chains and preserve the integrity of the electron transport train (ETT). As the first line of defense against free radicals, enzymes need to be supplemented in a balanced and synchronized way with pH enhancers to ensure enzyme activity.

We will talk more about the importance of pH in the following chapter, but for now, suffice it to say that when stress, toxins, or an acidic pH lower our levels of antioxidants, free radicals can damage our cells, and no part of the body is immune to their destructive effects. Protective barriers are breached in the intestines, and more toxins are absorbed into the liver. The result is that free radicals flood our bodies, running wild as molecular predators that attack cell membranes and DNA.

In their attacks on cell membranes, free radicals shoot deep inside cells, damaging the nucleus, which carries DNA, the genetic code of the cell. When they find their way to DNA or the mitochondria (the cell's energy factory), the free radicals rip electrons from them in their effort to stabilize themselves, causing cellular damage or mutations. (See Figure 4.1 on page 40.) Oxidative damage to DNA in humans occurs at a daily rate of about 100,000 hits per cell, reducing cellular energy, and playing a significant role in carcinogenesis.

Free Radicals and Aging

If allowed to continue their molecular terrorism against DNA, free radicals have the potential to do permanent DNA damage. Because our aging processes and life spans are controlled by our DNA, damage to our DNA can result in accelerated aging. In addition, when DNA is damaged, cancer cells can develop, multiply, and grow rapidly.

When proteins in the chromosomes of the DNA have been mutilated and deformed by free radicals, they accelerate degeneration and aging in the human body, especially in the brain and nervous system. Fats and proteins located on the cell membrane, however, help prevent neural and brain degeneration.

Special proteins called "G proteins" are held in their positions on the cell's membranes by phospholipids, a remarkable fat complex critical to hormone reception and activity. G proteins react to signal-bearing hormones by changing the cell's behavior. Let me explain briefly: A healthy cell membrane is like a telephone switchboard where signals from hormones or biophotons are either stimulatory or inhibitory, whichever is required to maintain balance in the body. G proteins act like an operator answering many calls simultaneously and diverting them to different extensions, regulating the flow between incoming signals and receptors, and determining when and for how long signaling pathways are turned on or off.

When phospholipids are rendered deficient by free radicals, G proteins become distorted and malfunction. When cell membranes are damaged, cells lose their ability to communicate with one another. Despite the presence of hormones in the bloodstream, receptor sites of cells fail to receive their messages. Most important, when cells fail to communicate with one another, they become inefficient at vital regulatory routines that keep us youthful, healthy, and full of energy. Alarm-reaction hormones (adrenaline and cortisone) damage the function of G proteins, resulting in disease. Obviously, we must do all we can to limit the damage of free radicals.

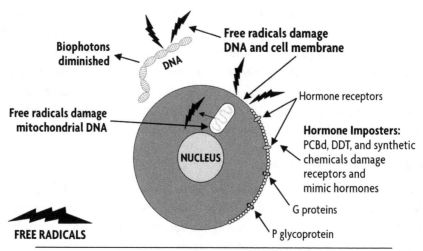

Biophotons
diminished

Free radicals damage
DNA and cell membrane

DNA

Hormone receptors

Free radicals damage
mitochondrial DNA

NUCLEUS

Hormone Imposters:
PCBd, DDT, and synthetic
chemicals damage
receptors and
mimic hormones

G proteins

FREE RADICALS

P glycoprotein

FIGURE 4.1. DNA instability and hormone receptor instability as pollutants
cause free-radical induced damage and mimic or block hormones.

Nutritional Antioxidants

As I mentioned above, oxidative stress initiates powerful chemicals that promote pain and inflammation in the body, as well as carcinogenesis, or the begin-
nings of cancer. In addition, nutritional deficiency leads to disturbed mitochondrial energetics, genetic alteration of mitochondrial DNA, and increased
exposure to mitochondrial carcinogens.

However, we can do something to prevent such occurrences. Optimum
food combinations can provide healing and rejuvenating energies to our biological systems with a 10- to 100-fold increase over less healthful foods in the
transfer of optimal energetic patterns. Indeed, in the year 2000, Jerome B. Block,
M.D., of the UCLA Medical Center in Torrance, California, presented data from a
number of valuable controlled scientific studies, all of which supported cancer
risk reduction with the use of antioxidants!

Repair to damaged DNA can be accomplished through antioxidant nutrients
that function as electron donors. They specifically protect DNA and cell membranes against oxidative damage, including that induced by carcinogenic agents.

While DNA repair mechanisms generally can repair the damage of occa-
sional exposures to oxidative stress, unrelenting damage to DNA can occur in
our bodies over our lifetimes. Protecting DNA with natural antioxidants, cellular
membrane phospholipids, and energy-enhancing nutrients and foods, therefore,
is critical for helping to stop faulty DNA-transcription of proteins.

Sadly, the average American diet does not always provide such protective substances. Rather, it often contains "foods" that can actually be injurious to our health.

FOOD THAT FAILS US

The unfortunate truth, however, is that what passes for food today is not only depleted of vital antioxidants, trace minerals, and phytochemicals but also contains harmful levels of pesticides and other toxic chemicals. Studies have documented that antioxidant levels in foods have decreased by 50 percent over the past twenty-five years in our great country.

The progressive depletion of antioxidants in food means that the majority of us live in an imbalanced state of excessive oxidative stress that may increase our risk of cancer. Indeed, studies have shown that diet accounts for 35 to 80 percent of cancers. Whole food, grown in organic, nutrient-rich, and chemical-free soil, provides the body with a synergistic array of thousands of known and unknown antioxidants, nutrients, powerful plant compounds, and light energies. These plant-based antioxidants help the body to counteract oxidative stress while simultaneously maintaining DNA stability. Assuming that these foods are pesticide-free, harvested in season, and appropriately prepared, they provide the best source of full-spectrum protection against oxidative stress.

Millions of Americans are faced with an ongoing daily battle with oxidative stress generated by worldwide pollution. These pollutants damage the cell's membrane and the cell's protective coating of phospholipids, thereby weakening the immune system. They can also block the QEF and reduce blood circulation by inducing red blood cell deformities. Boosting antioxidant enzyme defenses and providing the body with protective phospholipids may help to maintain cell membrane integrity and ward off viral infections.

With environmental carcinogens on the rise, our need for antioxidants has doubled, and then tripled since 1970. The consequences of this vis-à-vis cancer are the most telling. Instead of winning the war against cancer, statistics show we are facing a dramatic rise in the incidence of cancer and other chronic and degenerative diseases in the United States. In 1970, one out of fifteen people died of cancer. Today, one in three people die of cancer.

So far, we have looked at the body's own healing powers in its battle against stress and pollutants, and the role of food and nutrition in supplying antioxidants and repairing the body's systems. Next, we turn our attention to pH balance, and you can take the "Body Balance Test" to check your own balance and assess your "Alarm Reaction" to external stress and everyday toxins.

5

pH for Health and Energy

Optimal health may be characterized as being disease-free, injury-free, and highly energized, in other words, able to counteract attacks from pathogens, viruses, and other bodily stressors.

When too many toxins accumulate in your body, vital functions become disturbed, and your immune system may not be able to win the battle against infectious agents. Toxins can cause your brain chemistry to become unbalanced, causing fuzzy thinking or changes in your moods, thoughts, feelings, and behavior. Because it causes metabolic extremes, toxicity can actually incline us toward negative health habits, which create the basis for negative feelings and behavior of one kind or another. For example, people who suffer depression due to toxicity often crave foods that can lead to obesity. Or their depression can cause them to engage in a high-anxiety lifestyle in order to avoid exploring their feelings.

Detoxification, however, can be activated and maintained by exercise and nutrients that function as *cofactors* and *precursors*. A cofactor is a nutrient that must be present for a given chemical reaction to take place. A precursor is a nutrient that is needed for your body to produce additional nutrients that are critical to the detoxification process. (For example, thyroid hormone cannot be produced without the precursor iodine and the protein tyrosine.) But in order for these nutrients to be processed efficiently and to do their job effectively, the bodily "terrain" must be hospitable, *in balance*. What exactly, though, does "in balance" mean, and how do we go about achieving it?

ACID AND ALKALINE

Let's start with the continuous action of two opposing forces in the body: acid and alkaline. To maintain a healthy body, we need to maintain a particular *pH*, that is, a certain ratio of acid to alkaline in our system. According to leading medical physiologists, the balance of pH, which influences the orchestration of hormones and metabolic processes, is the single most important factor in the maintenance of good health.

You can measure your own pH by using pH tape (readily available at most pharmacies) dipped into your first morning urine or saliva. By matching the color on the tape to the accompanying chart, you ascertain your pH (see the Resources section for further information).

The pH can range from 4.5 (acid) to 8.0 (alkaline). For adults, the optimal pH ranges between 6.8 and 7.4.

pH and Nutrients

Like a tightrope walker who balances by making continuous adjustments, the reciprocal, mutually balancing action of various minerals helps to maintain the stability of the entire body by either stimulating or inhibiting bodily functions. Some minerals are acidic; others are alkaline. An excess of one mineral may be as bad as a deficiency of another mineral. A deficiency of only one mineral, such as calcium, can undermine the health of the entire body. Phosphoric acid is the predominant acid-generating mineral, whereas calcium, potassium, magnesium, and sodium are alkaline minerals.

When the body is too acidic, the function of all bodily systems becomes diminished. Our healing and repair mechanisms function more slowly and less efficiently. If it takes you a long time to get over a cold or flu, or to heal a cut, or if your doctor tells you that you are experiencing a degradation of your bones (osteoporosis), it could be an indication that your body is too acidic.

Foods can be either acid-forming or alkalizing. For example:

Some acid-forming foods:	Some alkalizing foods:
• cereals	• fruits
• eggs	• legumes
• fish	• potatoes
• fowl	• vegetables
• meat	• white flour
• nuts	• whole grains (except millet)
• sugar	

Our research has shown that to keep our QEF in balance, we need to eat 75 percent alkalizing foods and 25 percent acid-forming foods. Yet, the majority of Americans have diets consisting of 70 to 80 percent acid-forming foods! This unhealthy diet typically throws our blood sugar and hormones out of balance and depletes our QEF.

pH AND THE CYCLES OF STRESS

All kinds of stress tend to acidify the body by stimulating the manufacture of acid-producing chemicals and compounds. Eating too many acid-forming foods when we are under stress increases the depletion of the minerals calcium, potassium, magnesium, and sodium. This creates both biochemical and energetic imbalances that cause paralyzing fatigue and debilitating illnesses. Prolonged, unexplained fatigue often is found to be caused by a chronic deactivation and depletion of minerals and hormones, leading to a depletion of the QEF.

Not everyone responds in exactly the same way to the pressures of life. Some of us are able to rise above crises, while others are left devastated. Much of our ability to cope during, and rebound after, stressful life passages has to do with our overall state of health. Some clues to your own stress level may be found by reviewing your habitual behaviors, as well as the messages that your body is sending you. As a check on your body balance, take a few moments and take The Body Balance Test on page 46.

THE ALARM REACTION

If you feel tired when you get up, and then spend the rest of the day trying to raise your energy level with caffeine, nicotine, soda, megavitamins, sugars, and sweets, your body is in a state of alarm, owing to a hormonal imbalance.

How do our hormones get out of balance? As an example, I'll use an all too common phenomenon. A great many of us eat too many simple carbohydrates and sugars, things like breads, pastas, and snacks, such as commercial crackers and cookies. This provokes the pancreas to release the hormone insulin, the sugar-regulating hormone. Excessive insulin causes your blood sugar to drop too low, creating a stress reaction and stimulating the pituitary gland to produce a hormone called ACTH, which stimulates the adrenal glands. The stress-fighting adrenal glands respond to the pituitary and the threat of low blood sugar by producing adrenaline and cortisone, and these hormones set off an Alarm Reaction (illustrated by Figure 5.1 on page 47).

When excessive amounts of adrenal hormones are produced, an array of internal processes—such as circulation, respiration, digestion, and the secretion

The Body Balance Test

To easily check your stress levels, read the following items and check the ones that apply to you. Then read below to interpret the results.

Do you generally:

- crave starches and sweets?
- fail to eat a good, healthy breakfast?
- eat pasta daily?
- drink juices, soda, or other sweet drinks?
- need a cup of coffee or tea to get going every morning?
- eat margarine in place of butter?
- tend to eat low-calorie meals and drink diet sodas?
- eat fried foods daily?
- binge on sweets more than once a week?
- feel tired late in the afternoon
- feel sleepy after dinner?
- find it's hard to stay focused at work?
- frequently get headaches?
- frequently feel light-headed?

- yawn a lot during the day?
- feel depressed or sad once a week or more?
- suffer from allergies?
- wake up tired in the morning?
- feel nervous and irritable?
- drink any alcoholic beverages daily?
- have trouble falling asleep?
- wake up in the wee hours of the morning unable to sleep?
- have difficulty losing weight?
- have low sexual energy?
- have difficulty remembering things?
- have periods of anxiety?
- frequently get constipated?
- experience muscle pain or spasms?
- have low or high blood pressure?

If you answered "yes" to more than six of these questions, you could very well be experiencing some of the negative effects of stress. If you've answered "yes" to more than twelve of these questions, stress is seriously affecting the quality of your life. Your pH is very likely registering on the acid side, and your hormones are out of balance. Your body is in a perpetual distress cycle.

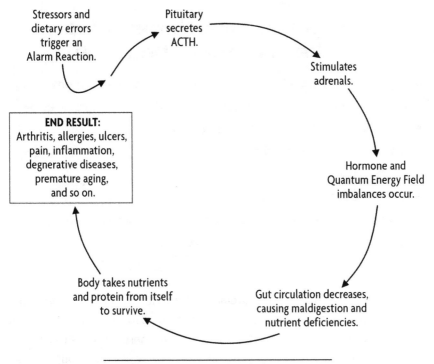

Stressors and dietary errors trigger an Alarm Reaction.

Pituitary secretes ACTH.

Stimulates adrenals.

END RESULT:
Arthritis, allergies, ulcers, pain, inflammation, degnerative diseases, premature aging, and so on.

Hormone and Quantum Energy Field imbalances occur.

Body takes nutrients and protein from itself to survive.

Gut circulation decreases, causing maldigestion and nutrient deficiencies.

FIGURE 5.1. The Stress-Induced Alarm Reaction.

of other hormones—becomes impaired. Our bodies enter a vicious cycle of accelerated aging and dysfunction.

Why our hormones can have such a detrimental effect on us can best be understood by considering the response to the threat of bodily harm or severe distress. Adrenal activity is directly related to our daily dietary patterns and stress levels. When we are confronted with real or seeming emergency situations, the "fight or flight" response of the adrenal glands prepares us by giving us a quick, short-lived blast of energy that speeds up our nervous system response and shifts the hormonal activity of the entire body into an alarm response reaction. When this occurs at an *appropriate* time—for instance, in a truly life-threatening situation, like a mugging or a shark attack—it can be life-saving. But when adrenal responses occur at *inappropriate* times, we become inappropriately aggressive, time-urgent, anxious, and paranoid. When our everyday diet sets off a "fight or flight" response because of dietary deficiencies or excess stimulants, we become hormone-depleted, unbalanced, and chronically stressed out. We become more prone to addictions, and in advanced stages of

Foods and Substances That Evoke the Alarm Reaction

Many modern foods and substances evoke in us an alarm response:

- foods high in trans-fatty acids, such as refined oils and margarines
- foods high in cooked, saturated, animal fats
- foods high in simple starches
- foods high in sugars
- foods or beverages high in caffeine or alcohol
- foods or beverages high in fruit sugars (fructose) or corn syrup
- foods that are over-processed or overcooked

this stress cycle, we may assume overactive lifestyles with hectic work schedules, turbulent personal affairs, and a tendency to dangerous and violent behaviors. As we continually provoke emergency responses from our adrenals—through inappropriate die—the ensuing stress cycle weakens our QEF and rapidly depletes our bodies of vital nutrients. Painful emotions, such as anger, grief, frustration, and fear, become all too common, and these only serve to fuel the cycle more aggressively.

When we stop overstimulating our adrenals, when we adopt an *appropriate* diet, we can break the vicious cycle of the Alarm Reaction, and gain energy, feel stronger, become more focused, and lead a happier life. We will also be able to recover from acute episodes of stress more quickly and without a loss of energy and stamina.

To control our stress response, lose weight, and live long and healthy, we need to eat lots of fruits and vegetables. Research shows that plant foods, packed with phytochemicals, can boost immunity, burn fat, and protect our bodies against disease. Let me make the point by telling you Andrea's true story.

Andrea's Diet Merry-Go-Round

Metabolism is the biological process by which energy (measured in calories) is extracted from the foods consumed, producing carbon dioxide and water as byproducts for elimination. Biochemically, this process involves hundreds of enzymes that are commonly deficient in the standard American diet. Energetically, metabolism involves the coordinated actions of all our bodies' meridians and their related organ functions to ensure that food is digested and assimilated for use. If the energy levels (as measured by the QMSM) are too low, than bioenergetic or physiological function will be low. If our pH is already too acidic, the stomach will not produce its own acid. It is the stomach's acid that stimulates other digestive organs to produce bile and pancreatic enzymes.

Rather than being burned in the metabolic process, calories will be stored as fat. In other words, it's not so much that "we are what we eat," but rather that "we are what we digest and assimilate."

Andrea was a fifty-four-year-old office manager of a large corporation, a very stressful position. Always on the run, she typically drank three to four cups of coffee for breakfast, frequently skipped lunch, and ate a late dinner, often consisting of the meats and fatty foods she felt cravings for, having starved herself all day. She complained of anxiety, indigestion, insomnia, and a loss of libido. On top of all that, she was thirty pounds overweight.

Testing the pH levels in Andrea's urine and saliva, we got a reading of 5.0. (If you recall, an optimal pH range is between 6.8 and 7.4.) The constant stress and poor diet had made Andrea's body too acidic, and she had a chronic depletion of the nutrients needed to produce and activate digestive enzymes.

To counter these problems, as well as her weight problem, we introduced Andrea to a program of quantum nourishment. Instead of her usual gallons of coffee for breakfast and no lunch at all, Andrea began to eat the Quantum Foods described in Chapters 10 and 11. After only two months of treating her body to real nutrition, Andrea's pH level was a much healthier—measuring 8.5—and she had lost twenty pounds! Clearly, her digestion was much improved, and even her anxiety and insomnia had been eliminated. And, at the end of the day, she reported "having energy to spare."

What can we learn from Andrea's story? Most often, when we gain weight, we assume that the answer is to eat less. As Andrea discovered, the real answer can be to eat more—of the *right* things. Proper nourishment leads to proper digestion. Calories are burned more efficiently. If you suffer from heartburn, flatulence, bloating, constipation, or loose stools (not diarrhea), it is a safe bet that you are not digesting your food efficiently, and the reason is most likely to be that you are not eating foods that organize and energize your QEF.

pH, ENZYMES, AND ENERGY

Many of us today are functioning in a state of near exhaustion. Our typical response to this condition is to stimulate—"energize"—ourselves with caffeine-containing beverages and sugar-laden foods. But as already observed, artificially stimulating the body when it is already in a fatigued state will eventually deplete one's QEF and lead to fuzzy thinking, sexual impotency, and a host of so-called age-related disorders.

As stress increases in the workplace and at home, more people are complaining of an "energy crisis." The effects range from what we've come to think of as "normal" fatigue, like listlessness, to premature aging and degeneration.

To create energy, the body uses two forms of raw materials: oxygen and food. As the oxygen enters the blood via the lungs, it is converted into the fundamental fuel of life, molecules called adenosine triphosphate (ATP). ATP is the source of molecular energy we need in order to function, maintain our youthfulness, and think intelligent thoughts. But in order to convert oxygen and food to ATP, we need enzymes.

An enzyme is a large protein molecule, containing vitamins; trace minerals, such as zinc, magnesium, selenium, and manganese; and other nutrients. A deficiency in just one trace mineral can have far-reaching ramifications. A zinc deficiency alone, for example, can render more than 120 enzymes dysfunctional.

Enzymes are also pH sensitive. When the body is too acidic, many enzymes fail to work at all or, in some cases, to work too much, making the body sick.

Without a daily dietary intake of enzymes from raw foods, raw food concentrates, and/or fungal-free digestive enzymes (99 percent of all digestive enzymes on the market contain harmful residues of fungus that only serve to stress your digestive system even more), none of us receives the optimum nourishment. In order for the body to maintain enzyme function, about 25 percent of each meal should consist of foods that are neither processed nor excessively heated. These raw foods ideally should be alkalizing foods that aid hormonal function. So which foods are most likely to serve our purposes?

The deceptively simple answer is, plants.

Plants get their energy directly from the sun. We derive the highest amount of our energy by eating plants (alkalizing foods) that are loaded with enzymes. Eating animals (acid-forming foods) that have eaten plants puts us lower on the energy food chain, so to speak. We receive less of the energy our bodies need to produce hormones, and raise the acidity of the body, as well. If we eat too much animal protein, the body can run short of energy-producing nutrients, leaving us exhausted, depressed, and unable to accomplish all that we desire. Nutrient shortages can also lead to an inability to think clearly, to sexual dysfunction and to a host of age-associated diseases, such as diabetes, heart disease, arthritis, and cancer. But by keeping your pH balanced and your QEF replenished with quantum foods, you can help stave off such disorders.

When you are low on energy, don't reach for quick-energy, acid-forming foods and beverages. Do not even consider even one of those commercial "healthy" power bars. Although these foods and beverages give us a "lift," there is also a direct negative effect on the body's hormone-producing glands and a depletion of your QEF. For example, the pancreas, which produces insulin, overworks every time we eat these stressor foods, and too much insulin throws all other hormones in the body severely out of balance. So begins the cycle of fatigue: While these foods provide temporary relief from physical or mental fatigue, they ultimately only drain us of more energy, affecting not only our health, but also our ability to enjoy life. Soon, the fatigue returns, and the cycle continues.

pH AND OXYGEN

Many cellular processes, including cellular energy production and healing, are fueled by oxygen. And the blood is most highly oxygenated when the body's pH is optimal. In a low oxygen, or anaerobic state, the immune system becomes disabled and the transfer of energy by way of biophotons dwindles. Without a properly balanced pH, acidification of the cell's external environment promotes oxidative stress, and healing levels of oxygen that are delivered to various parts of your body are decreased. While in a normal healthy person it should take only minutes for the immune system to restore itself after an incident of stress, one study published in the *Journal of Clinical Immunology* found it took *hours* for restoration, when the sedentary lifestyles of subjects resulted in reduced oxygen levels.

THE IMPORTANCE OF HEALTHY DETOXIFICATION

The biologic process of detoxification, that is, the body's ability to eliminate waste and potentially harmful toxins that accumulate in it over the years, is central to all bodily systems, especially a well-functioning immune system. Allergic individuals or individuals with ongoing or recurring yeast, fungi, or viral infections have faulty detoxification abilities. In fact, believe it or not, *all* immune and hormonal disorders involve deficiencies in the body's detoxification systems.

Hormones are the chemical messengers released by the endocrine glands. They are key to slowing allergic reactions, boosting immunity, stopping pain, reducing inflammation, and improving digestion. So important is the formation of hormones that scientists have formed a new field of medicine called intra-crinology devoted to studying this aspect of our health. Intracrinologists have discovered how key nutrients are necessary to trigger the formation of hor-mones, stimulate their activity in the body, and understand their effects on stress and the aging process. Interestingly, they have found that the same pre-cursors and cofactor nutrients used in detoxification also play a role in hormone production.

The liver is the vacuum cleaner for the blood. The liver's ability to detoxify the blood and produce hormones depends on enzymes and an adequately bal-anced pH. The pH and chemical balance of your detoxification systems deter-mines their efficiency and thereby the quality of your health, including your emotional health. When you empower your detoxification capabilities with the correct foods and supplements, you'll experience peak mental, physical, and emotional performance.

If your detoxification systems are working effectively, your body will rapidly be able to neutralize harmful environmental chemicals that you ingest from your air, water, and food supply, as well as those you absorb from social hygienic or from cosmetic substances you put on your body, such as soaps, shampoos, deodorants, or nail polish.

A Detoxification Caution

With the rise of pollution worldwide, detoxification methods are enjoying a renewed popularity, whether highly personalized and supervised by a health specialist at one of the world's elite spas, or completely do-it-yourself with a commercially packaged product purchased at the local health food store. Yet most people do not realize that some common products—as well as practices, such as fasting, coffee enemas, and colonic irrigation—can deplete the body's QEF and nutritional status even more than the impurities they are meant to get rid of. It's true. Unless you correct your pH and replenish your nutrient precur-sors and cofactor nutrients necessary for the liver to detoxify your body, these so-called detoxification methods only increase your chemical stress levels and/or toxicity. Alternative health practitioners will typically tell you that the "crisis" symptoms of fasting are "natural" and "normal." However, when your pH and nutrient levels are corrected and your QEF is balanced, there are no such reactions. Detoxification occurs *without further stressing your body.*

The only true gauge of the success of any detoxification measure is the percentage of toxins that are actually neutralized by the liver and excreted into the intestines. Unfortunately, many detoxification methods drive toxins out of the kidneys and into the bloodstream or lymphatic system and not into the bowels. When toxins overload the kidneys, people typically complain of skin rashes and itching, headaches, back and shoulder pain, chronic fatigue, and a host of other symptoms. The key is correcting your pH and QEF balance; then your body will detoxify without stress. Still, detoxifying the body alone is not sufficient.

Eliminate Everyday Toxins

It is important to understand that you must detoxify not just the body, but also the environment. Most households contain toxic chemicals used for cleaning or pest control. Get rid of products made with poisonous or otherwise hazardous materials such as insecticides, drain cleaners, and household cleaning products. Avoid exposure to toxins in personal care products, especially scented products and perfumes that are petrochemically based. Beware of solvents, like acetone, in nail polish and nail polish removers. Examine the ingredients in your cosmetics and be sure they are not toxic. If the ingredients are not listed, or the manufacturer will not disclose them, avoid the product.

The Appendix contains a list of common household and personal-care products that contain toxins linked to negative health effects. I urge you to make every effort to rid your home of as many of these as possible.

Needless to say, it's also critical to end the willful or habitual ingestion of toxic substances. Thus, we recommend that you kick toxic habits, such as smoking and heavy drinking; avoid eating fast foods; do not consume any processed or hydrogenated fats; and avoid drinking coffee and sodas, all of which stimulate and suppress the QEF. Finally, do not ingest toxic supplements. Note that 97.6 percent of supplements currently available are toxic and increase detoxification burden on the liver.

Besides avoiding dangerous things, there are positive steps you can take to improve your health. For example, you need to drink eight to ten glasses of hydrated and energized water daily. Hydrated water is purified and specially treated so that it is actually wetter and can penetrate the cells and tissues more effectively.

Last, but by no means least, exercise at least thirty minutes every day, and get at least fifteen minutes of sunshine, three times a week. This combination of exercise and sunshine, in combination with a healthy diet, protects you from a range of ailments, from depression to bone disease and even tooth decay.

6

Environmental Toxins: The Dangers and How to Avoid Them

While normally quite adaptable and resilient, our bodies are also perhaps the most delicately tuned "machine" on earth. Their intricate functioning is affected not only by lifestyle stresses and the foods we eat, but also, both positively and negatively, by numerous factors and substances in the environment.

ELECTROMAGNETIC FIELDS (EMFs)

One hundred years ago, life in the country was full of fresh air, clean water, and rich soil. The energy of the sun and the earth's magnetic frequencies were naturally resonant. Now, however, due to innumerable factors, including overpopulation, deforestation, and personal and corporate pollution, this environment has slowly been degraded and contaminated. Today, a very serious problem is the proliferation of electromagnetic fields (EMFs). During the past ten years, as satellite-controlled cellular phones and television and computer satellite links permeate the air and our bodies with 60-cycle frequencies and other anticoherent energies, technology based EMFs have increased dramatically.

EMFs permeate our bodies' QEF through our acupuncture points, adding more information to the interaction between the QEF and the cells of the body. The effect is like trying to listen to a radio station while several stations' signals vie for the same narrow strip of the band. The result is static with only intermittent clarity. In our bodies, the result is a lack of coherence, an internal imbalance, and an attempt to adapt to the stress. Unfortunately, such adaptation takes a toll on our health and vitality.

EMFs from electrical equipment and common household and office devices can continually throw off our bodies' equilibrium. They also upset the brain/ nervous system's control over tissues, organs, and systems of the body. Since the nervous system uses simple, nonlinear electrical patterns to maintain homeostasis, it is extremely sensitive to environmental frequencies that are similarly simple and nonlinear.

Concern over health effects from EMFs was prompted as long ago as 1979, when a 7 million dollar study by the California Department of Health Services showed how children who lived in close proximity to electrical lines had a greater than 50 percent probability for childhood leukemia, as well as risks for adult brain cancer and Lou Gehrig's disease. In addition, it suggested a 10 to 50 percent possibility that EMFs could increase the risk of male breast cancer, childhood brain cancer, suicide, Alzheimer's disease, and "sudden death."

POLLUTION AND ENVIRONMENTAL ESTROGENS

There is mounting evidence that human exposure to chemicals, even at low levels, can be harmful. Such exposure is linked with adverse biological effects, including endocrine disruption, chemical sensitivity, delayed healing, prolonged infections, and cancer. Lifetime exposures can cause irreversible injury to the body.

According to world-renowned authority on quantum physics, Dr. Fritz-Albert Popp, toxic chemicals act as biophoton light scramblers. For example, during wartime, communications are kept from an enemy by using devices designed to scramble messages, thereby creating confusion and misinformation. Biophoton scramblers act in an identical manner, causing DNA instability and disrupting the communication of powerful streams of healing energies in the body.

Estrogen, naturally present in all of us, is a hormone that regulates many physiological processes, including growth and reproductive function. An *environmental* estrogen, sometimes called a *xenoestrogen* (literally "foreign estrogens," and also referred to as endocrine-disruptors, endocrine-modulators, ecoestrogens, and hormone-related toxicants) is a substance that *acts like* an estrogen hormone in living organisms. Exposure to environmental estrogens occurs throughout our lives, both from the food we eat, and also from household products, including detergents, drugs, aerosols, lubricants, dyes, cosmetics, pesticides, synthetic fabrics, and plastics. Direct exposure also comes from drinking water that has been contaminated by the chemicals and their toxic byproducts released into the water we drink by industrial discharge and sewage waste. We are also indirectly exposed when chemicals are released into the air and water, and when airborne fumes from industry or hazardous waste incinerators land on grass or hay and are eaten by livestock that is subsequently consumed by humans.

Protect Yourself from EMFs

EMFs are generated by all electrical devices (hair dryers, electrical outlets, telephones, and common household appliances, such as vacuum cleaners, microwave ovens, and garbage disposal units). In today's world, it is next to impossible and surely impractical to avoid using electrical devices. But there are a number of protective devices available that will convert EMFs into harmless energies.

Phone Protectors. The phone protector is simply a specially treated diode— a metallic conducting coil—that converts the specific EMFs from the telephone into biologically harmless energy. It's easy to install and never wears out. Simply stick it on to the back side of the earpiece of your phone receiver.

Cellular Phone Protectors. Like the phone protector, this diode is specifically designed to convert harmful microwave EMFs from your cell phone into harmless frequencies. Just affix it near the earphone receiver of your cellular phone.

Computer Protectors. Monitors emit x-rays, ultraviolet, and low-frequency EMFs. Like the EMFs emitted from a television screen, these radiations require four specially treated, hi-tech diodes. Simply place them near each corner of your monitor's screen. For laptops, these may be placed on the four corners of the back of your screen (the lid) so you are not prevented from closing your computer.

DC Protectors. These are specially designed diodes for battery-operated devices such as pagers, headphones, or watches. Placing one on the back of these devices eliminates all harmful EMFs.

Circuit Protectors. Circuit protectors neutralize EMFs in your home. Place one diode on one of the outlets on each floor and say goodbye to all harmful EMFs from household appliances.

See the Resources section for sources of these products.

Many of these xenoestrogens have been associated with developmental, reproductive, and other health problems in living organisms. And since they are stored in body fat cells, they adversely affect fetal development in a mother's womb and, later, infant development through breast milk.

Understanding Your Endocrine System

To understand the dangers of environmental estrogens to your health, you'll need to know the basics of how your body communicates with itself via natural hormones produced by the endocrine system. The endocrine system is a complex network of glands, such as the pituitary, thyroid, pancreas, and gonads (testes in men; ovaries in women). These glands control and regulate many bodily responses and functions, both immediate and ongoing, through the production of hormones. They work hand in hand with our nervous system to produce, use, and store energy; maintain the body's internal functions (metabolism, excretion, and water and salt balance); regulate growth, development, and reproduction; and react to stress and other stimuli from outside the body.

The hormones produced by the endocrine system carry messages to specific body parts about temperature changes, hunger, emotions, growth needs, or other stimuli. Hormonal responses can be speedy (as in response to fear) or they can react more slowly (as when they regulate growth and gender maturation).

These chemical messengers travel throughout the body, seeking out and locking onto special binding proteins, known as receptors, located in and on the cell targeted by the hormone. The receptor reads the hormone's message and carries out its instructions to affect growth, sexual and reproductive maturity, male and female sex characteristics (breast size, bone density, muscle development, and sperm production), cycles (uterine growth and pregnancy), and the regulation of blood sugar levels and heartbeat.

Among the many hormones produced by the endocrine system is estrogen. As you've learned, environmental estrogens, or xenoestrogens, act like a natural estrogen hormone in living organisms, but unlike natural estrogen, which stays in the bloodstream only for short periods of time, xenoestrogens accumulate in body fat or tissue and can block or mimic natural hormones for longer periods of time. This can destroy receptors, confusing the endocrine system's communication network. Xenoestrogens also deplete nutrients needed by the liver to detoxify the body and manufacture natural hormones, and they depress thyroid function, causing fatigue and weight gain, leading to increased pain and inflammation in the body.

Research has linked xenoestrogens to birth defects, autoimmune diseases, chronic conditions in children (such as attention deficit hyperactivity disorder, depression, and asthma), and chemical sensitivity, including its overlaps with sick-building syndrome. They have also been linked to the unexplained illnesses of Gulf War veterans (these have also been attributed to exposure to mycoplasmas), chronic fatigue syndrome, fibromyalgia, Syndrome X, neural degeneration, and cancer. Even allergies and recurrent infections have been linked to accumulations of environmental estrogens in the body.

Many of these chemicals are lipophilic, meaning they gravitate toward fat molecules rather than water molecules, congregating in fatty tissue and staying there for years. When we have been exposed to these estrogenic chemicals, our bodies will attempt to flush them out, but many will be absorbed into the body where they collect (or bioaccumulate) in fat and muscle. Repeated exposure, without healthy detoxification, can lead to serious illnesses in later life. Reproductive system failure can occur decades after the exposure to and subsequent buildup of these toxins in the body. As we get older, our bodies tend to collect and store more and more of these synthetic compounds. During stress, pregnancy, or breast-feeding, these substances can be released from fat and redistributed or passed on to offspring.

Strong evidence of the threat posed by xenoestrogens appeared in a study published in the *Journal of the National Cancer Institute,* where researchers reported that xenoestrogens increased the incidence of cancer by 400 percent.

How Xenoestrogens Alter Hormonal Functions

The xenoestrogens in our endocrine system alter our hormonal functions by:

- **Mimicking** or partly mimicking the sex steroid hormones estrogen and androgen (the male sex hormone) by binding to hormone receptors, thereby altering the cell's normal functions;

- **Blocking, preventing,** and **altering** natural hormonal binding to hormone receptors, thereby interfering with the body's sensitive and delicate internal communication system;

- **Decreasing** the production and breakdown of natural hormones; and

- **Modifying** the production and function of hormone receptors.

Xenoestrogens and Wildlife

Researchers have also found that xenoestrogens (pesticides, industrial chemicals, and other pollutants) are responsible for reproductive abnormalities in wildlife. In his book *Our Stolen Future,* Theo Colborn reported that male Florida alligators became feminized after a severe pesticide spill; male fish living downstream from sewage outfall produced a female hormone; and tadpoles living in pesticide-ridden waters had between zero and 67 percent deformities, versus zero and 7.7 percent deformities for frogs in noncontaminated waters.

High levels of contaminants found in wildlife document that living creatures store and accumulate these substances just as humans do. One environmental study showed that samples of wildlife blood contained DDT concentrations of 1 milligram per milliliter, a level about 1,000 times higher than concentrations of natural estrogens in blood. Several studies have found that even polar bears, seals, and humans living away from industrialized areas in the relatively pristine Arctic have significantly elevated levels of many different pesticides and industrial waste products.

Despite more than forty years of credible research on xenoestrogens, and the extinction of animal species reported in areas where they were exposed to these toxic elements, the chemical industry has mounted a campaign to discredit researchers who have reported the negative effects of xenoestrogens on animal and human populations.

Thus, for some, profits are more important than prevention. That being the case, what can we do as individuals to limit the impact of such substances?

Checking Labels: Common Xenoestrogens to Avoid

Xenoestrogens are causing a worldwide epidemic of chronic illnesses as, among other things, they inhibit natural healing. Reducing our exposure to them, by whatever means we can, is of the utmost importance. Yet every day we eat them, drink them, breathe them in, and use them at work, at home, and in the garden. They are present in soil, water, air, and food and are increasing at an alarming rate. The fact is that environmental estrogens are everywhere and can't be completely eliminated. But by maintaining our pH balance and boosting the health of our bodies' natural detoxification systems, we can protect ourselves. In addition, by refraining from the use of the household and personal-care products (many are listed in the Appendix), we will reduce the load of these toxic chemicals in our bodies. A partial list of dangerous chemicals can be found in the inset on page 61.

Harmful Pesticides

Begin by assuming that all pesticides are harmful, as they contain large amounts of xenoestrogens. Avoid spraying your lawn, garden, or home with pesticides, and throw away all pesticides (insecticides, herbicides, and fungicides) that have one or more of the following chemicals on the label:

- Alachlor
- Aldicarb
- Atrazine
- Benomyl
- Chlordane
- Dibromochloropropane
- Dieldrin
- Dichlorvos
- Dicofol

- Endosulfan
- Ketone
- Mancizeb
- Methoxychlor
- Nitrogen
- DDT
- Phthalates
- Toxaphene
- Tributyl tin

In addition to discontinuing use of these products, try to minimize your exposure to them by avoiding foods that you know have been grown with the use of commercial pesticides.

Another common source of xenoestrogens is solvents that are commonly found in nutritional supplements, cooking oils, laundry detergents, fabric softeners, and cosmetics such as nail polish and nail polish remover. Paints, varnishes, and a wide spectrum of household cleaning products are loaded with solvents. Here are the most common ones to look out for:

- Alcohols such as methanol;
- Aldehydes such as acetaldehyde;
- Esters, commonly referred to as ethyl acetate;
- Ethers, commonly referred to as ethyl ether;
- Glycols (propylene glycol and ethylene glycol);
- Halogenated hydrocarbons (carbon tetrachloride and trichloroethylene);
- Hydrocarbons (hexane, benzene, and cyclohexane);

- Ketones (acetone and methylethylketone); and

- Nitrohydrocarbons, commonly referred as ethyl nitrate.

The effect of the above chemicals are additive and synergistic, which means they are strengthened when used together. Researchers have documented that, in combination, they are thousands of times more toxic than when exposure is to a single chemical.

Personal body-care products also contain xenoestrogens and potential carcinogens. Every time you use a xenoestrogen ingredient on your skin, you alter and suppress your QEF. Here is a list of the most common ingredients to look out for:

- **Fragrances.** Many synthetic fragrances (not the real herbal or plant scents) are toxic petrochemicals (petroleum-based chemicals) that enter the body quickly through the skin and accumulate in lipid-rich tissues, such as the brain and nerves, and fat tissues of the body.

- **Parabens.** These chemicals (propylparaben, methylparaben, butylparaben, or ethylparaben) are cheap synthetic preservatives used to inhibit microbial growth in nearly 99 percent of all cosmetics. However, parabens also promote excess viral activity in your body.

- **Sodium lauryl sulfate (SLS).** This is a harsh, caustic detergent used as an engine degreaser and garage floor cleaner. It is commonly found in body soaps, shampoos, and facial cleansers. A potentially dangerous mutagen, SLS is capable of doing serious damage to your DNA.

- **Mineral oil.** Petroleum-based mineral oil clogs your skin pores and interferes with the ability of your skin cells to eliminate wastes and absorb nutrients.

- **Imidazolidinyl and diazolidinyl urea.** Commonly used as preservatives, these substances release formaldehyde, which is a powerful xenoestrogen.

- **Propylene glycol.** This is a powerful xenoestrogen used as an emulsifying base in creams and lotions to make the skin look smooth. It denatures the skin, blocks meridian energy flow, and is potentially toxic to your liver and kidneys.

- **Synthetic colors.** Artificial tints are used to color cosmetics and are commonly labeled as FD&C or D&C, followed by a number and a color. (Henna, as a natural plant-based dye, is an exception.)

OTHER ENVIRONMENTAL CONCERNS

We live in an age of genetically modified (GMO) and chemically treated foods and supplements. Do these pose any danger? In 1989, a genetically engineered dietary supplement, L-tryptophan, took the lives of thirty-seven persons in the United States alone. Another 1,511 cases of a syndrome known as eosinophilia myalgia syndrome also have been linked to this supplement. In 1990, the journal *Science* documented the fact that a toxic, genetically produced amino acid found in this dietary supplement was attacking the immune system, making joints ache uncontrollably, and causing limbs to become swollen.

Genetically engineered foods and modern agricultural farming methods are depleting our soil and food of nutrients needed by our bodies to protect themselves from environmental assaults, especially viruses.

A number of events could trigger massive epidemics worldwide. For example, we know that infectious disease is affected by changes in the weather. With the "El Niño" effect, warmer winters will no longer "freeze" the spread of infection as colder winters once did. Thus, global warming has consistently been linked with an increase in infectious diseases and deadly viruses, especially in recent years.

Since the 1970s, environmental stressors have caused a dramatic increase in cancer and disease rates, and experts have estimated that more than half of the population will become chronically ill and incapacitated in the next decade. Modern medicine has been less than responsive, leading almost 40 percent of Americans to seek help from alternative medical practitioners. Mainstream healthcare providers have been stunned at the complexity of pollution-generated illnesses. They come up empty-handed for effective medications, or even for reasonable explanations as to why people have become ill. Sooner than most doctors and scientists can imagine, allergic, inflammatory, and hormonal disorders will double and triple in the general population. The illusion that modern medicine has things under control will be gone, and with it, the quick-fix drug solutions.

TAKING STEPS

We must all ask ourselves, Am I at risk from increasing worldwide pollution? Is my body presently capable of excreting and neutralizing these harmful chemical invaders?

Take a moment to revisit the list of stress-gauging questions in Chapter 5. (See "The Body Balance Test" on page 46.) If you answered "yes" to more than twelve of the questions, you've most likely accumulated substantial amounts of environmental estrogens in your body. In fact, you are probably *"estrogen dominant,"* that is, your hormones are out of balance. In addition, if you have difficulty dealing with ordinary stress, losing body fat, or functioning sexually, it could mean your body is overloaded with these estrogenlike toxins.

It's critical that we begin now to adopt a sensible diet to replenish the nutrients we have lost over the years. Be sure to read labels for chemical ingredients, and avoid genetically modified (GMO) foods. Adopt the healthy eating habits that I will explain in greater detail in Chapters 8 through 11.

Nature's Healing Foods: Phytochemicals

In the 1980s, the U.S. Department of Agriculture estimated that 185 million acres of American farmland were eroding at more than twice the rate at which soil can be replaced naturally. Dr. Bernard Jensen, in his 1990 book *Empty Harvest,* documented the widespread demineralization of our soil, the declining nutritional values of our food supply, and the resultant weakening of our bodies' immune systems.

The foods we consume are extremely complex mixtures of bioactive constituents that work together to nourish the human body. Our metabolism and immune systems function best with antioxidant (free-radical fighting) and enzyme-rich foods consumed in their natural, raw state. When our intake of fresh fruits and vegetables is too low, our bodies' ability to counteract daily assaults from our toxic environment is weakened.

The unfortunate fact is that the overwhelming majority of American foods not only are depleted of vital antioxidants, enzymes, trace minerals, and phytochemicals, the importance of which I will be discussing shortly, but they also contain carcinogenic (cancer-causing) chemicals. The prolonged consumption of such foods leads to cancer.

Although the stunningly complex molecular puzzle that underlies carcinogenesis remains incomplete, parts that seemed unrelated a decade ago now seem to be fitting into place. Research has documented that carcinogenesis can be counteracted by the antioxidant power of whole foods.

FOOD ADDITIVES, CONTAMINANTS, AND TOXINS

The foods typically consumed by the general public every day are far from pure. They contain dozens, if not hundreds, of additives. Despite the fact that many of these food additives have been found to be carcinogenic or mutagenic in laboratory animals, they are continually used in a wide array of processed foods, because "experts" proclaim that they have never been tested and proven detrimental to *human* health! Faced with the vast number of additives now used in commercially manufactured foods, regulatory agencies must wait for established evidence of toxicity on humans before they can insist that these be removed from food products. For example, added colors or dyes are found in cereal products, baked goods, snack foods, meat, fish, poultry, cheese, butter, and other dairy products, and alcoholic and soft drinks with the average individual's consumption estimated at 100 milligrams per day.

Mycotoxins (toxins found in molds and fungi) increase the risk of liver cancer, and because they stress the immune system, they can contribute to carcinogenesis; more than 300 different mycotoxins have been reported in foods and animal feeds. In fact, in 1985, the Food and Agriculture Association estimated that 25 percent of the world's food crops are contaminated with mycotoxins. High levels of mycotoxins were reported in peanuts, tree nuts, cereals (grains), beans, and apples. More than a dozen studies citing the high carcinogenicity of mycotoxins in animals were reported by the Institute for Cancer Research. Supplements, especially fungal-derived digestive enzymes, also contain high levels of immunosuppressive mycotoxins that increase one's risk of developing fungal infections. In fact, in our own clinical research on digestive enzyme products, we found only two out of fifty products that were pure and completely free of remnant fungal (aspergillus) residues.

Heterocyclic amines, or HCAs (ammonia derivatives containing more than one type of atom) found in grilled meats and fish are responsible for high mutagenic activity. If your diet is high in animal protein, you are undoubtedly exposed to excessive HCAs. Studies now show that short-term feeding (six to twelve weeks) of HCAs is enough to induce tumors in experimental animals. Accumulation of HCAs has also been linked in human studies to a higher occurrence of colorectal cancer than in control subjects.

While numerous individual potential toxins have been studied, one major limitation of research on additives and human cancer risk is that there have been no studies to assess the effects of the *combination* of thousands of food additives consumed together in our food and drink. This effect may be even more toxic than the sum of individual additives that have so far been looked at in animal studies.

IS "NATURAL" BETTER?

Chemical additives are found in virtually all manufactured foods and drinks, even in so-called "natural" products. In the mass manufacture and distribution of processed foods at prices people can afford, the food industry frequently resorts to processing techniques that degrade the plants' original health-promoting nutrients. Some who are aware of the deficiencies of processed foods may try to avoid these, but it's far from simple. For instance, while organic food may be richer in minerals and antioxidants than commercially grown food, many organic farms are located in highly polluted areas and/or use contaminated water to irrigate their crops. Not surprisingly, these carcinogenic agents filter into the soil along with acid rain and alter the natural nutrient content of organic foods.

As a result, significant levels of carcinogenic agents may be found even in these presumably healthier foods. So "natural foods" are better, but that depends to some degree on your definition of "natural." Thus, in addition to identifying and eliminating specific carcinogens in the food and drink we consume and in the body-care products we use, daily supplementation with pure, raw, whole, unprocessed foods supplements is of critical importance in preventing carcinogenesis.

PHYTOCHEMICALS TO THE RESCUE

Over the last several decades, industrialization and urbanization have meant that fewer people are growing their own food or even buying it locally grown. This has resulted in a dietary shift from being predominantly plant-based to one that is typically animal-based. This is significant because plant-based foods are rich in phytochemicals (*phyto* meaning "plant" in Greek), powerful compounds that plants produce to protect themselves from excessive sun exposure, disease, and insects. In consuming plant-based foods, we absorb a wide variety of bioactive phytochemicals, which function as protectors of our inner and outer cellular world, and have been shown in studies to inhibit carcinogenesis. According to David Heber, M.D., Ph.D, Director of the University of California, Los Angeles, Center for Human Nutrition, "There are about 25,000 [different kinds of] phytochemicals in the world, and we're finding that they perform special functions in the cells to help prevent diabetes, common forms of cancer, heart disease, age-related blindness, and Alzheimer's disease." It seems obvious that we need fewer chemical additives and more natural *phytochemicals*.

Fighting Free Radicals with Phytochemicals

Part of our own bodies' natural defense system is the production of antioxidant chemicals and molecular compounds that counteract free radicals before they cause damage to our cells.

As you've learned, a free radical is an unstable and, therefore, toxic oxygen molecule produced as a natural byproduct of our metabolism. But *excess* free radicals are caused by innumerable stressors, such as cigarette smoke, x-rays, air pollutants, and food additives. Uninhibited, they are capable of destroying cells and glands that produce natural hormones.

Many phytochemicals function as antioxidants. They stabilize free-radical oxygen molecules, delaying, inhibiting, or preventing their damage. Phytochemicals also are powerful pH balancers that improve the efficiency of hormone transport and regulation throughout the body. A diet and supplementation program high in phytochemical-rich fruits and vegetables is important to overall good health. However, it's important to be aware that phytochemicals lose their potency when food is cooked, processed, or grown in polluted environments, and they are destroyed at temperatures over 118°F. So food preparation can be just as important as choosing the right foods. Most methods of cooking and processing leave food devoid of phytochemicals.

Fighting Cancer with Phytochemicals

A diet rich in antioxidants, that is, a diet containing fresh fruits and vegetables, has been shown in 128 out of 156 dietary (epidemiological) studies to be protective against cancer. According to Jerome Block, M.D., of UCLA Medical Center, ". . . there is sufficient pertinent, scientific, clinical data to indicate that certain antioxidant and other nutrient supplements reduce cancer risk, clinical cancer occurrence, and/or interrupt the carcinogenic process in appropriately-defined populations."

For those already dealing with cancer, for whom prevention is not the primary concern, Mark C. Houston, M.D., and John A. Strupp, M.D., of Vanderbilt University School of Medicine, had this to say about reducing the toxic effects of chemotherapy: "A judicious, scientifically-based use of supplements would not only make the patient feel better subjectively, but would reduce complications, promote surgical healing, reduce infections, possibly reduce the growth of a tumor, prevent metastasis, and allow the oncologist to use higher doses of chemotherapy and radiation when needed, without increasing complication rates."

Plant foods that contain abundant quantities of these substances, such as *lycopene* from whole, fresh tomatoes, *carotenoids* from fresh carrots, and *glu-*

cosinolates and isothiocyanates from raw broccoli, have consistently been shown to be associated with a lower risk of cancer at almost every site of the body, and studies show that they activate critical detoxification enzymes that decrease the bioavailability of potential toxins or pollutants, that is, they obstruct DNA-damaging carcinogens. They also boost critical antioxidants needed to facilitate the destruction of toxins into innocuous, excretable substances.

Boosting Your QEF with Phytonutrients

Phytonutrients are plant-derived nutrients, far superior to synthetic or man-made vitamins or soil-derived minerals because they are biologically active and easier to digest and assimilate into our cells. Scientists are finding significant relationships between our hormones and phytochemicals in the food we eat. These powerful youth-generating compounds provide the body with nourishment needed to increase the production of natural anti-aging hormones. Phytochemicals sharpen the mind and boost the body's metabolism, resulting in more muscle and less fat. These powerful plant extracts and compounds promise to extend the human life span and give us a chance to live a full, productive, and more youthful life. Imagine being able to maintain the peak hormone levels or immunity of a twenty year old as you grow older.

In that phytochemicals organize and strengthen the body's QEF, phytochemical-rich foods provide state-of-the-art nutrition for boosting immunity; losing weight; fighting allergies; enhancing physical, mental, and sexual performance; resisting viral infections; and tempering your body's response to stress.

Clinically, I have found a consistent association between accumulated toxins and a reduction of the body's QEF. Proper nourishment—consisting of the appropriate phytonutrient, herb, and phytochemical combinations—can activate your body's remarkable ability to cleanse itself, eliminating built up toxins, and slowly move the body in the direction of peak performance and vibrant health.

Phytochemicals and phytonutrients found in fresh, uncooked plant food can take you beyond the benefits of ordinary vitamins and beyond ordinary energy, vigor, and resistance to disease.

Faced with many enzyme-depleting stress factors, millions of people in their forties and fifties really need a daily intake of phytochemicals in order to function optimally. But it is important to recognize that phytochemicals are not the same thing as multivitamin supplements taken by more than 40 percent of Americans. Synthetic supplements often *interfere* with the body's natural cycles of hormone production, allowing hormone-producing glands to weaken and atrophy from disuse. Phytochemicals, on the other hand, do not supplant glandular function; rather, they restore youthful levels of hormones by providing the body with the raw ingredients needed to *manufacture* and *maintain* adequate levels of hormones itself.

Empirical and groundbreaking research in the field of Quantum Medicine has shown that:

- Phytochemicals and phytonutrients can *inhibit* cancer, and

- Phytochemicals can *increase* cellular levels of antioxidants and cause the body to neutralize and excrete toxins.

Further phytochemical research and technology promise to prevent a wide range of modern-day illnesses.

8

Combating Viral Infections and Mycotoxins

Viral threats to our well-being and survival have increased immeasurably. While most of us survive these daily threats without noticeable ill effects, damage is still occurring. By the time symptoms have appeared, however, they can often be difficult to reverse. The good news is that the response of the immune system can be enhanced and maintained, allowing us to cope effectively with these stresses and prevent them from causing illness.

Immunity involves all systems of the body in a dynamic interplay, which enables the body to recognize foreign invaders and neutralize and/or metabolize and eliminate them. Guiding and empowering this multifaceted response is the intelligence of the body's QEF.

In order for the immune system to properly identify an invader, it must integrate information from the QEF. This energy field is constantly scanning our internal and external environment for dangerous organisms or chemical toxins. When operating efficiently, this surveillance system orchestrates the immune response with the other systems of the body into a harmonious and unified whole of great power and precision.

One system in particular, the digestive system, serves two critical and immunological functions: It provides a protective barrier and defense against infection, and also supplies nourishment to the immune system and all the cells of the body. We take the digestive system for granted, for the most part, but it is actually quite complex—and proper nutrition even more so. To illustrate, let me tell you Jason's story.

JASON'S BATTLE

Jason, age forty-five, had suffered for more than a decade with chronic fatigue syndrome (CFS). Doctors were unable to offer any solutions to his endless fatigue, chronic headaches, digestive problems, allergic reactions, and insomnia. An endocrinologist prescribed cortisone and antibiotics, but none of these drugs improved his condition. Jason was resigned to living with less energy, but the quality of his life had been greatly diminished.

Jason's blood tests with the endocrinologist revealed borderline low levels of thyroid hormones; all other tests fell within the normal range. His doctor told him that overall these levels were normal for someone his age, that he did not need hormone replacement therapy.

Jason read all he could about nutrition. He avoided junk foods, ate natural foods, and took vitamins. He even consulted with an alternative health practitioner who diagnosed a chronic viral infection, Epstein-Barr virus, and prescribed natural remedies. Despite all of these efforts, Jason's symptoms remained the same.

Finally, Jason heard about Quantum Medicine and consulted a certified doctor. Jason's physician prescribed bioactive peptides, which function as natural enhancers of human growth hormone (HGH), a proteinlike hormone naturally secreted by the pituitary gland. All body systems—regulation, regeneration, and cell replacement—depend on HGH. But studies show that HGH production declines after the age of twenty at a rate of 14 percent per decade. By sixty years of age, it is not uncommon to measure a HGH loss of 75 percent or more.

Jason's doctor also prescribed raw coconut butter as a superior way to boost steroid hormones like DHEA (as DHEA increases, it also increases the production of HGH), testosterone, and powerful phytochemicals to restore DNA.

Quantum nourishment, consisting partly of phospholipids and bioactive peptides, improved Jason's liver function, causing his HGH levels to increase dramatically. Jason's DHEA also increased slightly. In only four weeks, Jason reported a complete disappearance of all his symptoms. He felt supercharged with energy.

The vitamins and hormones that Jason previously had taken were synthetic. And though he ate natural foods, he did not eat them in the correct balances. He had been drinking raw carrot juice, and eating excessive amounts of sweet fruits and grains, which, because Jason was extremely hypoglycemic, triggered an Alarm Reaction in his adrenals. Every time he ate excessive amounts of these foods, he blocked hormone production and activity. Unknown to his endocrinologist, Jason's chronic headaches had been caused by the enlargement of his pituitary gland. When the adrenals and thyroid gland are too weak to respond, the pituitary gland fatigues and swells. This is the cause of many chronic headaches. In most cases, underactive adrenal and thyroid gland function precede states of pituitary dysfunction.

After two months on the Quantum program, Jason's blood tests revealed that his HGH and thyroid hormones had returned to normal levels, and his chronic viral infection was no longer a threat to his immune system.

It should be noted that without knowledge of the intricate web of inter-dependent, overlapping, and complex functions of other systems of the body, HGH replacement therapy may produce no health-enhancing or anti-aging effects. While one study reported favorable results with HGH replacement ther-apy, other studies reported side effects and no improvement of the pituitary gland.

Based on inconclusive evidence, it appears that diet and nutrition is the preferred method of enhancing this powerful hormone.

The natural dietary and nutritional enhancement of HGH works by halting the Alarm Reaction, freeing up the liver to do its job of removing and inacti-vating gonad hormones. When HGH is optimal, patients report improved lung capacity, decreased body fat, improved cardiac and kidney function, and stronger immunity. Improved testosterone or estrogen levels are results of this therapy.

CHRONIC FATIGUE AND THE QEF

Chronic fatigue syndrome (CFS) has become a common disorder in primary health care. Although Epstein-Barr virus has been implicated as one of the caus-ative factors, medical experts lack definitive diagnostic and therapeutic tools for assessing and treating CFS and lack effective antiviral therapies. Our own clinical studies, as well as several other studies, however, point to a state of hypoxia (lack of oxygen) and acidity in patients with CFS. One study done with an electron microscope found cellular deformations, deficiencies in micro-circulation, and deprivation of oxygen in CFS patients.

These studies, then, indicate that chronic states of exhaustion and fatigue result from overworked and undernourished endocrine glands. When hormones are out of balance, the body works harder, using more energy to accomplish its regular functions, and the QEF is depleted.

With diminished QEF, victims of CFS experience delayed, slowed, or exag-gerated responses to many biological events in the body. This regulatory slug-gishness causes both time and energy to be wasted in responding to stimuli, and thus, the principles of energy conservation and homeostastis—the chemical balance within both cells and organs—are upset.

Circulation is the primary means by which the neurohormonal system maintains homeostasis. Any disturbance in blood flow will produce the regulatory deficits that result in chronic fatigue. In addition, since less oxygen means less energy, reducing acid states and promoting increased oxygen with a quantum energy-based diet is integral to the success of alleviating chronic fatigue.

A deficiency of alkaline minerals such as magnesium is also a common finding in cases of chronic fatigue. One study documented that CFS patients have lower magnesium levels and that treatment with magnesium improves energy and emotional status.

In addition, the importance of proper adrenal function also cannot be overstated. When overstimulated, the QEF and adrenals become compromised and are then unable to provide the body with an optimal immune defense.

When the body is in the unhealthy alarm state, it excretes excessive amounts of adrenal hormones that bring on indigestion. This, in turn, disturbs the healthy balance of intestinal bacteria (flora) and inhibits the detoxification functions of the liver. This results in infection, which could be fungal or yeast (Candida), Epstein-Barr virus (EBV), or bacterial (strep). Indeed, as studies show, there is a high incidence of undetected infections in people who are ill. In one study of 7,148 patients, a group of doctors reported a high incidence of chronic infections in their patient population.

The vicious cycle of fatigue, illness, and infection can be halted when nutritional therapy is directed at reestablishing hormonal balance and the open flow of energy through the acupuncture meridians of the QEF. The adrenals then function optimally, digestion improves, and chronic fatigue is eliminated.

NEW WEAPONS IN THE WAR AGAINST VIRAL THREATS

In addition to our general concern about viruses, we have, regrettably, acquired an additional cause for concern regarding these infectious agents: Terrorists, as well as our own military, have been experimenting with engineered viruses that may not respond to medical treatment or vaccinations. But we actually can protect our bodies from viral plagues by understanding the way viruses infect the body.

New insights gleaned from the human genome and from antiviral research conducted by the pharmaceutical industry have been nothing short of breathtaking. The advanced antiviral research of pharmaceutical companies provides some additional clues we may follow as we attempt to learn how to aim anti-infective agents at viral infections on multiple levels, instead of aiming treatment at a single phase of viral activity.

Despite these advances, drug researchers admit to one serious flaw in the clinical potential of their findings: Viruses develop drug resistance or insensitivity to treatment and can mutate at lightning speed, so that drugs fail to provide effective long-term treatment and immune protection. Pharmaceutical research also tends to look for a magic bullet to target only one phase of viral activity, failing to consider the broad role of the QEF in antiviral responses by the body.

To combat novel viral strains, we must understand thoroughly the mechanisms that viruses use to gain entrance to target sites in a host (body) as well as the strategies that the body uses to prevent them from doing so.

How Viruses Attack Us

As a result of much ongoing research, we have learned that:

- Viral infection spreads when the pH of our cells is too acid or too toxic;

- To infect cells, viruses take advantage of nutrient deficient cell membranes or excesses of trans-fatty acids;

- Viruses can enter the cell more efficiently when free radicals have damaged the cell membranes;

- Each virus attacks a particular type of cell (for example, cold viruses attack the lung's cells; the AIDS virus attacks the T4 cells of the immune system).

In other words, in order to replicate and do damage to the host organism, viruses must invade living cells. Once a virus is able to attach to a receptor on the cell membrane, it can then penetrate the cell. Strategies to enhance the immune system against viral invasion must be designed to enhance the immune system's ability to patrol, enforce, and attack invading microbes with greater efficiency or operational complexity by reestablishing quantum coherence.

Once in the cell, the virus sheds its lipid or protein shell. Then it effectively hijacks the cell's genetic material and makes a DNA copy of its own genome, which it then inserts into the host cell's DNA. Because viruses use the same basic mechanisms for subjugating cells (this can vary slightly depending on the type of genome the virus possesses), they can crank out copies of viral DNA at incredible speeds in the nucleus of the cell. Whatever its genome, a virus is capable of producing millions of new viral particles with the aid of the cell's raw material and machinery. While some viruses act only at their point of entry (adenoviruses, for example, invade the eye causing conjunctivitis), others move beyond their point of entry and spread through the lymphatic system, causing a generalized infection of many tissues of the body that later erupts into a full-blown infection when stress overwhelms the body.

Quantum Medicine's Defense against Viral Infection

In my search for a natural way to implement the new discoveries of drug researchers, I have uncovered a unique combination of herbs, phytochemicals, and phytonutrients that can nourish the body's army of immune cells that identify, tag, blast, and consume invading microbes. This unique antiviral approach takes into account, for the first time, the extraordinary complexity of the immune system at the quantum level as it stores information and establishes communication with the entire organism faster than the speed of light.

In the quantum approach to protection, natural compounds are combined that simultaneously can bar viral entry into the cells, jam the copier to halt viral replication, improve DNA coherence and stability, stop viral traffic, and halt the spread of infection throughout the body. The clinical goal was to target and strengthen specific organs or glands of the body via the selective uptake by the various tissues of the body of phytochemicals and fermented mycelial extracts (medicinal mushrooms).

In acknowledging the weblike interaction and interpenetration of the immune system with all other systems of the body, especially the human energy system, a quantum antiviral strategy capitalizes on the immune system's vastly superior qualities to fight its own battles.

Despite the reductionistic tendencies of mainstream medical research, Quantum Medicine has provided us with important pieces of the antiviral puzzle. Let's examine some of the major highlights of this research:

- **Medium chain fatty acids (MCFAs).** Some studies have suggested that ingesting MCFAs can reduce viral load by 50 percent by uncoating lipid-enveloped viruses before they enter cells. The best medium chain fatty acid we know of is coconut butter, discussed more fully in Chapter 10.

- *Viscum album* (mistletoe). Rich in glycoproteins, polypeptides, lignans, and triterpenes, *viscum album* has the unique ability to stabilize genetic mechanisms at the quantum level, resulting in quantum coherence. Studies have suggested that by normalizing DNA, *viscum album* is capable of actually reversing cancer at the biophoton level.

- *Larrea tridentata* (chaparral). Scientific studies have documented the powerful antiviral activity of this unique and powerful plant; it is a potent and aggressive lymphatic cleanser, able to detoxify the lymphatic system and eliminate viral infections.

- **Fermented mycelial extracts.** Our research has found that for immune enhancement and bioregulation against viral infection, effective mycelial extracts are produced by fermenting the mycelia part of the *Hericium erinaceus, Grifola frondosa, Reishi, Ganoderma lucidum,* and *Cordyceps sinensis* mushrooms and combining these with tissue- and organ-specific phytonutrients.

An effective viral defense, therefore, depends on following some basic nutritional protocols:

- Maintaining pH and healthy detoxification (as discussed in Chapter 5);

- Complete dietary elimination of trans-fatty acids (margarines, processed cooking oils, and genetically modified oils such as canola oil) because viruses thrive and seem to penetrate deeper into the body when these fats are in the daily diet;

- Maintaining DNA stability with appropriate antioxidants from phytochemicals (as discussed in Chapter 7);

- Supplementation with nutrients critical to the health of cell membranes;

- Immune-enhancement strategies that establish quantum coherence and penetrate all dimensions of the immune system.

Hence, effective antiviral agents must be able to penetrate into the lymphatic system, helping lymph nodes and other immune centers of activity to function with greater operational complexity and strength.

The overwhelming majority of natural immune-enhancement approaches fail to prevent the viral entry into the cell and the viral hijacking of the cell's unstable genes, because they fail to consider the critical role of quantum coherence in the design of their approaches. The cell-to-cell spread of the virus can be prevented or stalled by augmenting immune responses with appropriate phytochemicals. However, all phases of viral infection must be targeted for optimal results.

Effective immune-enhancement therapies must be multidirectional, that is, not push the body too much in any single direction. In addition, it is imperative that all immune responses be fully supported and maintained in order to subdue and conquer viral invaders and speed recovery from viral infection.

Bear in mind that the complex interactions of the immune system are primarily powered by biophotonic events. Like an orchestral conductor bringing each individual instrument into a beautiful, collective sound, biophotons work individually, and yet harmonize together to achieve quantum coherence. And the better the coherence between these communication events in the sub-molecular world of cells, the greater power the immune system has in preventing and counteracting viral overload. When quantum coherence is reestablished at the genetic level, our immune response may be so fast and effective that we may not even be aware of a viral invasion.

The ability of viruses to wreak havoc should not be underestimated. Since viruses can swap genes or parts of genes, new viruses are constantly emerging, or known viruses can evolve into a form the immune system cannot recognize. Hence, viral mutations and/or genetically engineered superbugs impose serious and even lethal threats to the human body. Nutritional deficiencies contribute to this concern by reducing the integrity of the cells and their processes, allowing viruses to enter cells and trigger mutations. Identifying and correcting deficiencies, therefore, should be undertaken without delay.

New molecular technologies are helpful in understanding new generations of viruses and in developing new strategies to outwit deadly forms of new viruses. While more research is needed to document these theoretical ideas and clinical insights, it certainly appears that by reestablishing quantum coherence and using multidirectional immune-enhancement techniques, we may be able to increase survival rates against some of the world's deadliest viruses.

MYCOTOXINS AND TREATMENT RESISTANT SYNDROMES

While much attention lately has been given to the dangers associated with stealth infections, it's surprising that the dramatically increasing health threat of mycotoxins—secondary metabolites produced by many species of fungi—is still being largely overlooked. Mycotoxins are naturally occurring chemicals that are produced by fungi growing on feed, food, or grain. These fungal metabolites are highly toxic and highly suppressive of the immune system. Unfortunately, they are increasingly present in processed foods, especially in peanuts, tree nuts, beans, apples, grains, and cereals. In 1985, The Food and Agriculture Association estimated that 25 percent of the world's food crops are contaminated with mycotoxins, and the number is probably much higher today.

According to the World Health Organization, mycotoxicosis can cause Alzheimer's disease, multiple sclerosis, atherosclerosis, and cancer. In addition, many studies have documented that mycotoxicosis is a causative factor in multiple chemical sensitivity syndrome, as well as respiratory and neurological disorders. The research of Iris R. Bell, M.D., of the University of Arizona Health and Sciences Center, showed abnormal brain-wave activity among patients exposed to mycotoxins. Bell and her fellow researchers documented that mycotoxins have a direct biological role in initiating and/or perpetuating nervous system–related illness. The connection between the environment and health, according to A. V. Constantini, M.D., from the University of California, School of Medicine, San Francisco, is not that major diseases are caused by the consumption of specific foods, but that they are caused by the fungi and mycotoxins present in the food chain.

IRRADIATED FOODS: A CURE WORSE THAN THE PROBLEM?

Food irradiation, which ostensibly kills bacteria and gives food a longer shelf life, has a decided downside, one that negates any so-called benefits of the process. Irradiation in foods causes an overgrowth of deadly strains of mycotoxins that disable the liver and cripple the immune response.

Since September 11, 2001, the practice of irradiation has become even more widespread, in an effort by authorities to kill viral strains such as anthrax. Foods, homeopathic products, and nutritional supplements are being irradiated with electron beams that are a hundred million times stronger than the beams passed over carry-on luggage at the average airport security checkpoint x-ray. Electron beaming penetrates cell walls and stimulates oxidative stress. It breaks down DNA, scrambles or "unfolds" proteins, and inactivates enzymes in foods and supplements. In destroying food's molecular structure, potential nourishment is likewise destroyed. So the effect is dually deadly: food loses its sustaining and healing benefits, and also harbors illness-producing agents! In addition, when we irradiate foods that contain fats, we create other byproducts called *cyclo-butanones*, a class of extremely toxic radiolytic (radioactive) chemicals that have been documented to cause genetic and cellular damage to human and rat cells.

Born out of a fear of terrorism, as well as pressures from the 460 billion dollar food-processing industry, irradiation is on the rise. Missing from consideration is the fundamental principle of public health: If, in order to make food safe to eat, you destroy nourishment, you destroy health. One problem is that when food is irradiated, it *looks* the same; what is forgotten is that the destruction is at the cellular level. When vital nutrients that support the immune system are lost, and mycotoxins overload the liver, disabling its detoxification mechanisms, a simple virus can easily overpower the immune system and create severe and prolonged viral illnesses.

Why would the government permit irradiation to take place if it is so dangerous? Perhaps, it has been misled by much of the early public university research on food irradiation that it funded during the 1960s and 1970s, which was positive, but has subsequently proven to be inconclusive. It is obvious to me that we need to conduct new research—by objective scientists who will ask the right research questions.

Until that research is done, and we have clear evidence of the damage that irradiation causes, we need to eliminate irradiated foods and supplements from our diet altogether. Also, to reduce harmful solvents and mycotoxin levels, we should thoroughly soak all grains, nuts, legumes, and seeds prior to cooking or consumption. Since it is so difficult to determine what harmful processes commercial food products may have undergone, to the extent possible, we should avoid commercially processed foods, as well.

9

The Brain:
Our QEF Regenerator

All of our "vital organs" are interrelated and interdependent. We could not survive at all without a heart or a lung, for example. But concerning the *quality* of life, surely the brain is the most important. Yet it is also one we take so much for granted. In this chapter, we will examine the brain from the quantum health point of view—and take nothing for granted.

Healthy brain power is determined by three interrelated and interdependent factors: the chemical environment and physical structure of brain cells (called neurons); the efficacy with which the brain communicates with the rest of the body; and how well the brain manages and stores memory.

It takes a good part of our lifetime to achieve wisdom and gain knowledge, but, sadly, in our senior population, millions suffer from a severe loss of memory, rational thought, and the ability to communicate. Mental deterioration renders valuable life-gained wisdom unavailable when, in the last decades of our lives, we most need it. A lifetime of uncompensated stress that has upset the physical functions of the brain has relegated great numbers of seniors to nursing homes when they should be thoroughly enjoying their hard-earned "golden years."

In some individuals, the rate of mental decline is imperceptibly slow, while others seem to lose mental function suddenly and without warning. By making healthy choices, individuals can ward off brain disintegration (senility or dementia) and many age-associated signs of neural degeneration. The food we eat can nourish and protect the brain, or it can cause our memory and reasoning abilities to deteriorate.

Considering the high demands of modern-day living, how profoundly faxes, e-mail, and call waiting have increased the demands for our attention and added a lot more word- and idea-processing to our average day, it's easy to understand why a high percentage of people suffer from some degree of brain fog, memory loss, and forgetfulness. Even people who have not lost any of their mental acuity can experience intense distractibility on any physically and/or emotionally taxing day. Who isn't forgetful, at least once in a while?

It's been said that if you lose you keys now and then you are probably OK, but if you find your keys and can't remember what to do with them, you may have a problem. Certainly, if you lose your keys three times a day, there is a likelihood of something more involved than simple forgetfulness. Many so-called normal reactions to stress—poor organization, insomnia, procrastination, forgetfulness, insecurity, restlessness, and anxiety or depression—can, over time, progress into severe brain impairment.

In the wake of life stress, it is a tuned resonance between the heart and brain that is responsible for replenishing or regenerating our QEF via the flow of chi or prana—an energetic intelligence—between the two. When properly functioning, this heart-brain resonance interfaces with any blockage that has been caused by stress and vibrates those discordant, blocked energies out of the body.

As we begin to age, many of us find it harder to remember certain types of information, such as names, dates, addresses and phone numbers. Dull memory, lack of concentration, mental confusion, and other neurological symptoms are signs of brain aging and a loss of healing energies.

Our mental and physical health depends to a large degree on a state of internal balance between excitation and inhibition, and an overall organization and rhythm between the meridians and the brain. Disruption of this balance and rhythm is the primary cause of decreased mental performance.

NUTRIENT DEFICIENCIES AND NEUROTOXINS

Millions of adults and children diagnosed with attention deficit disorder (ADD) face the problems of coping with poor concentration and memory, finishing what they start, and organizing their lives.

Critical to the brain's proper functioning are *neurotransmitters,* hormone-like messenger chemicals that travel the pathways of the nervous system with information necessary for regulating both body and mind. A deficiency of only one nutrient needed to construct a neurotransmitter will impair our thinking and behavior.

In addition, just as there are xenoestrogens that pollute and stress our hormonal communication, there are *neurotoxins* that pollute and stress our neural communication. When these toxins enter the brain, they cause severe behavioral problems, confusion, hyperactivity, and an inability to perform more than one task at a time. Enzymes are needed to detoxify and excrete these neurotoxins.

The presence of neurotoxins in the body is actually a double whammy. They are, in and of themselves, damaging, but they also deplete nutrition at an incredible rate! Nutrient deficiencies cause an array of symptoms, such as poor memory, anxiety, depression, hyperactivity, and the symptoms of ADD. So faulty information processing is most commonly caused by a *combination* of nutritional imbalances and deficiencies coupled with toxicity in the brain.

Today, one in every six children in America suffers from autism, dyslexia, attention deficit disorder, hyperactivity, or aggression. According to the *U.S. News & World Report* of June 19, 2000, there has been a 210 percent increase in autism in California between 1987 and 1998, and a 55 percent increase in learning disabilities in New York between 1983 and 1996. A growing body of evidence suggests that neurotoxins are contributing significantly to these problems. A recent study from the National Academy of Sciences suggests that a combination of neurotoxins and genetic/DNA instability may account for nearly 25 percent of developmental problems in children, those who, because they are still growing, are particularly vulnerable to neurotoxins. Normal brain development and cell-to-cell communication may slow down, accelerate, or even be damaged by gaps in the brain's electrical wiring. Studies on neurotoxins at the State University of New York at Oswego showed that babies with *polychlorinated biphenyls* (PCBs) in their umbilical cords—due to the mother's exposure to these toxic chemicals—performed more poorly than unexposed babies in tests assessing visual recognition of faces, ability to shut out distractions, and overall intelligence. The problem in America is so profound that the U.S. Department of Health and Human Services is presently asking Congress for 1 billion dollars to track 100,000 children from the womb through high school to assess the effects of chemical exposure on childhood development.

We can illustrate the relationship between chemical exposure in children and their physical and mental development by telling John's story.

John's Struggle with ADD

John was a five-year-old child diagnosed with ADD. His mother's attempts to understand John's suffering were obvious, yet she was exasperated with what turned out to be futile efforts to control his behavior. When John took his prescribed Ritalin to "solve" the problem, he became withdrawn and passive. When his mother stopped the Ritalin and consulted another doctor, he suggested that food allergies might be involved, but this approach also proved unsuccessful. John's behavior and symptoms continued unabated. John also suffered from rashes, asthma, and sinusitis. While on antihistamines, cortisone, and antibiotics for these allergic symptoms, his behavior grew more hyperactive and bizarre.

When John was six, his mother brought him to a doctor who practiced Quantum Medicine. Extensive testing revealed that John had chronic nutrient deficiencies. The doctor also identified a dysfunctional liver that was essentially overloaded with neurotoxins, including synthetic cortisone. He believed John's extreme sensitivity to food additives also could be attributed to the high levels of neurotoxins.

But because John's liver had been rendered dysfunctional; he was unable to detoxify his body, and his enzyme levels were so low that he couldn't make sufficient neurotransmitters. Without enough neurotransmitters, the delicate balance between John's brain and his nervous system had been derailed.

An adequate intake of healthy foods and nutrients, the building material for enzymes, hormones, and neurotransmitters, can restore the critical balance between hormonal and neural events. New research has revealed that tiny cells of the brain and nervous system harbor amazing internal communication networks that operate through a process called *volume transmission.* By studying this brain transmission process, scientists have achieved revolutionary advances in understanding why and how the brain malfunctions. For the first time, targeting nutrition to enhance volume transmission has the exciting potential of speeding up the process of how *neurons* store memories and process information. Quantum nourishment means supplying the body with superior forms of nutritional complexes designed to infiltrate neurons, and provide the brain with the fuel it needs to send and receive messages from the body.

After only one month on Quantum supplements, John's mental and physical health improved dramatically, and his ADD disappeared altogether.

DHEA and Medium Chain Fatty Acids (MCFAs)

More than 150 hormones are manufactured by the adrenal gland. One of them, dehydroepiandrosterone, known as DHEA, is a powerful hormone that regulates a wide variety of key functions in the brain and body.

Steroid hormones such as DHEA and testosterone are depleted in many diseases, and the amounts produced by the body decline with age. For example, individuals in their eighties produce only 10 to 20 percent of the DHEA they produced in their twenties.

Since 1966, more than 5,000 scientific papers have appeared on DHEA, revealing a wealth of information and intriguing findings. There is, for instance, substantial research evidence that DHEA has the remarkable ability to repair brain cell damage, stimulate antioxidant enzyme production, and counteract the brain-aging effects of stress and viruses.

Supplementation with synthetic or even "pure" forms of DHEA, however, fails to strengthen weak adrenal glands and balance all of the other adrenal-produced hormones. Adding medium chain fatty acids (MCFAs) to one's diet is superior to hormone replacement/supplementation therapies, because MCFAs augment the healthy production of steroid hormones.

Found in raw, unprocessed, and unheated coconut butter, MCFAs, the "forgotten nutrient," is readily available. Although it has yet to receive a great deal of publicity in the media, it is the most important nutrient for the health of the brain and the QEF.

According to scientific research, MCFAs:

- Lower cholesterol and reduce the risk of heart disease, artherosclerosis, and stroke;

- Fortify cell membranes against free radicals and viral entry into cells;

- Help to clear out "bad" fats, especially trans-fatty acids and LDL cholesterol, to enhance steroid hormones and the QEF, via improved biophoton communication in the body.

Since heart disease has been linked to trans-fatty acids, it makes good nutritional sense to include MCFAs in your daily diet. So you should include raw, unprocessed, and unheated coconut butter in your daily diet to insure that you get sufficient MFCAs—for the health of your brain and your QEF.

Another "forgotten" substance is the hormone melatonin. Next, we examine the relationships among melatonin, light, the pineal gland, and health.

THE PINEAL GLAND AND MELATONIN

Melatonin is a natural hormone made by the pineal gland, which lies at the base of the brain. When the sun goes down and darkness arrives, the pineal gland goes to work, releasing melatonin into the bloodstream. As melatonin production rises, you begin to feel less alert. Your body temperature starts to fall, and sleep seems more inviting. With the coming of dawn, however, melatonin levels drop quickly to but a trace.

As far back as the 1800s, scientists linked mental deterioration with an abnormal pineal gland and low levels of melatonin. When pineal glands are removed, patients complain of depression, headaches, anxiety, and hallucinations, establishing a clear link between the pineal gland and healthy mental functioning. Numerous studies document how exposure to natural sunlight can improve the function of the pineal gland and brain.

In addition, in his 1950s book, Mark Altschule, M.D., of McLean Hospital in Boston, reported a high success rate treating mental states with nutrition. But what of the role of melatonin? Contrary to the belief of many mainstream and alternative health practitioners, there is no clinical evidence that melatonin supplements can restore the pineal gland's normal regulatory function. Johan Beck-Friis, M.D., found low levels of melatonin in people under severe emotional stress, and a group of university psychiatrists also reported low melatonin levels in depressed children. But these researchers focused only on melatonin and not on the additional factors of environmental stressors, such as neurotoxins. Taking melatonin may be helpful, but it only helps to replenish one deficiency of the pineal gland.

Light—sunlight, in particular—is integral for healthfulness. As I mentioned earlier, individuals with seasonal affective disorder (SAD) suffer from depression, low energy, food cravings, insomnia, low self-esteem, and feelings of hopelessness. In my own research, I had a group of patients blink into the sun twenty times a day for fourteen days, and I was amazed at the improvement in pineal gland function. In winter time, I had people with low melatonin work and read under full spectrum light bulbs (see the Resources section for further information). Again, the results were astounding. All of these patients were relieved of insomnia and other symptoms of a melatonin deficiency—without taking supplemental melatonin.

Lastly, as I discussed in Chapter 6, EMFs generated from computers, hair dryers, microwave ovens, and household appliances can disturb the delicate functions of the body. This is especially true with the pineal gland. (The Resources section provides product information on diodes to reduce the harmful effects of EMFs.)

Since a fully functioning pineal gland plays such an important role in our health—particularly in our sleep cycles and in mood regulation—it is important to do the following:

• Get natural lighting in your home or spend time in natural sunlight at least three days per week;

• Eliminate or neutralize any harmful EMFs in your bedroom and in your home environment.

STABILIZING DNA

Brain cells stiffen or harden when the body is too acidic or too toxic and depleted in protein and other nutrients. And, as we learned in Chapter 5, proteins in the nervous system become depleted by prolonged Alarm Reactions and hormonal responses to our dietary intake.

In addition, stabilizing our DNA prevents free radicals from damaging brain cells, especially the myelin sheath, the covering of nerve fibers that carry messages to and from the brain. This loss of nerve transmission is also accompanied by a stiffening of brain tissues and a disruption in volume transmission, which affects the speed and efficiency with which we process information (think) or retrieve information (remember).

When DNA is unstable, protein becomes mutated, causing many functions of the body to become impaired. As far back as 1853, the German pathologist Rudolf Virchow discovered in the cell's environment starchlike deposits of mutated proteins and amyloid, a hard protein deposit resulting from tissue degeneration. Later, it was discovered that the these aberrant or mutated protein complexes result in a decline of neurotransmitters; they also generate a complex and progressive cascade of molecular changes that distort cellular membranes, interfere with nerve transmission, and clog the cells of our bodies. We had found the basis of many forms of neurological disease.

When DNA is unstable, protein becomes mutated. This often leads to some form of dementia, even Alzheimer's disease (AD). We believe these destructive proteins overrun the brain, forming plaque in and around nerve fibers. These denatured proteins damage areas of the brain that control reasoning and memory. Thus, it comes as no surprise that a majority of people who have been diagnosed with AD have shown elevated levels of cortisol and adrenaline, the stress hormones that flood the body during an Alarm Reaction.

When enzyme activity is diminished and adrenaline and cortisol are too high, protein can stiffen the brain and nerve tissues. When the aged brain loses many neural pathways, reaction time is longer, memory is poor, and the learning process is impaired. Cellular responsiveness to hormones and neurotransmitters becomes diminished.

Premature brain aging occurs primarily at the cell membrane level. Damage to cell membranes is related to acidic pH, deficiencies in MCFAs, and cell membrane receptor malfunctions. Brain aging is also caused by free-radical damage, to which the brain is especially vulnerable because of its high use of oxygen.

The brain consumes one-fifth of the oxygen taken into the body. Brain cells contain fats, and these become rancid when oxidized; brain cells produce only low levels of antioxidants, and aged brain cells lack the multi-protective effect of MCFAs and DHEA. The fatty substances critical to brain cell function must be digested and assimilated from good and wholesome food sources. But unfortunately, as we age, the body's ability to break down fats into nutrients called fatty acids is reduced by as much as 50 percent. Nutrients must be presented in such a way that they can be easily assimilated by the brain cells.

Vital phospholipids, components of brain cell membranes, help to restore youthful nerve functioning and transmission of nerve impulses. These signal-enhancing nutrients also play a role in increasing the number of neurotransmitter receptor sites. Phospholipids combined with essential fatty acids provide the raw materials for increasing flexibility and cell membrane signal transduction, enhancing function even in the aging brain.

In this chapter, we have looked at the brain as an organ. We have been reminded that the brain, too, must receive nourishment, oxygen, and sunlight; that it, too, can have its nutritional deficiencies; that the proper functioning of the brain is dependent on the complex interplay of a number of vital substances, such as DHEA, MCFAs, melatonin, phospholipids, coconut butter, and more. In the next chapter, we will look at the Quantum Foods, those that will provide the brain and the rest of the body with the ultimate in nourishment and vitality.

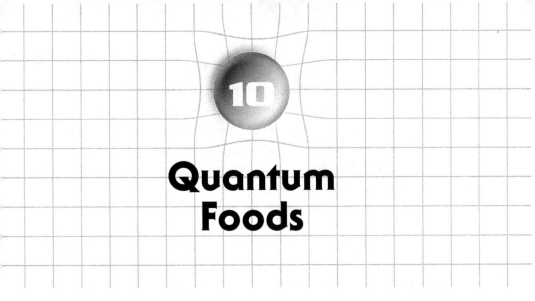

Quantum Foods

The eating habits of Americans leave a great deal to be desired. We tend to consume excessive amounts of acid-generating foods that lower the body's pH and block enzymatic conversion. Cooked animal proteins and highly refined and processed foods, American favorites, throw our pH out of balance and interfere with the metabolism and production of "good" eicosanoid (anti-inflammatory) hormones. We also consume a high percentage of deep-fried foods containing trans-fats, which retard hormonal activity. Most Americans eat for taste rather than for nutritional value. But many of us know that it's time to change those negative habits. We just need to choose what we consume according to new standards.

THE NUTRITIONAL VALUE OF FOOD

Overall, the most important aspect of the food we eat is its wholeness, by which I mean, the closer it is to its natural state—the less processing and/or cooking it has undergone—the more of its original nutrients remain intact. Four other factors also determine how much of the inherent nutritional value of a given food we will be able to absorb and use:

1. Quality

Finding high-quality food today is a challenge. Try to ensure that the food you buy is fresh. Avoid genetically modified (GMO) foods or foods that have been irradiated or sprayed with harmful chemicals to extend shelf life.

Since 1970, we have seen an astonishing 850 percent increase in the amounts of toxic chemicals in our food. These toxins are stored in the liver, spleen, and lymph nodes, and in the fat tissue of our bodies, so they accumulate over time and become more dangerous as they do so.

While irradiation may kill the bacteria that cause decay in food, this process also destroys food nutrients and produces radiolytic byproducts such as formaldehyde, benzene, formic acid, and quinines that cause free-radical stress on your QEF. GMO foods, moreover, are the *number one* enemies of your QEF, and they will undoubtedly create chaos in biophoton communication, disrupting your healing capabilities dramatically.

On October 18, 1999, *Business Week* reported, "Almost 60 percent of all processed foods in the U.S.—and virtually all candy, syrup, salad dressing, and chocolate—already contain GMO material." Since the U.S. Food and Drug Administration (FDA) does not require labeling of GMO foods, it's difficult to know exactly when you are eating them. By avoiding processed foods altogether and eating more whole foods, you can reduce your exposure to harmful GMO-treated foods.

2. Quantity

Even good food can overload the digestive system if consumed in excess. Overeating burns unnecessary energy, causes internal stress from maldigestion, and accelerates depletion of the QEF. A good rule of thumb is to eat no more at one time than can be held in two hands. Studies show that caloric restriction results in extended youth and longer life in test animals, retards aging of the pineal gland, and reduces sugars to levels that prevent glycation, stressed-caused damage.

Since it requires such sacrifice, most people do not succeed in making the severe cutbacks in the amount of food they eat, even though that would enable them to experience many long-term health benefits. The goal of the Quantum Energy Diet, therefore, is to consume more of nutrient-dense foods that are rich in the important healing compounds that *block* glycation without necessitating caloric reduction.

3. Enzyme Content

Enzymes are found in abundance in raw food and are easily destroyed by cooking and processing techniques.

According to reliable government statistics, loss of nutrients in our food ranges from 32 to 75 percent when the usual cooking methods are employed. New scientific research estimates that, because of depleted soil, as well as processing, even before we cook our food, it is already 50 percent depleted in antioxidants.

Research experiments with cats provides a valuable illustration. Cats fed pasteurized milk and cooked meat lost their teeth, experienced organ dysfunction, and developed arthritis; those fed raw milk and raw meat remained healthy with no trace of disease.

Other research, done by Paul Kouchakoff, M.D., of the Institute of Clinical Chemistry in Switzerland, has demonstrated that processed and cooked foods also have an adverse affect on the human immune system; they lower the white blood cell count, while raw, natural food do not.

4. pH

Alkaline foods are preferable to acidic foods and should make up 75 percent of the diet. Most fruits and vegetables are alkaline, while most grains and animal-derived proteins are acidic.

RECOMMENDED FOODS

In our search for those life-enhancing foods, we must keep in mind the four factors just mentioned—quality, quantity, enzyme content, and pH. When all four factors are combined, we then have superior nutritional value, as summarized in the inset "Food Recommendations" on page 92. Use it to guide your daily/weekly menu, household shopping, and food preparation.

UNLOCK YOUR HEALING POWERS—WITH FOOD

At every moment, energetic streams of life permeate every molecule of our bodies. It is this life energy that maximizes the functions of the organs and systems. Our dietary choices have consequences. We are aware that toxins and substances such as cholesterol plaque can build up in our arteries and veins, choking off the vital supply of blood and nourishment to parts of our physical bodies. Likewise, certain food substances can create blockages in energy flow that choke off our healing capabilities.

Through the foods we consume, we can either enhance this energy or we can disrupt the natural flow and create disturbance and depletion of our QEF. When consumed, the nutrients of whole, fresh, raw foods add to our own energy field and increase our potential for healing. By changing your diet in keeping with the findings of Quantum Medicine, you hold the power to transform meals into an opportunity for healing.

The following are some simple, practical, energy-enhancing eating strategies that I encourage:

- Supplement your diet with Quantum Foods described in the next chapter. These superior foods are far above the quality of any organic food you can buy in your local health food store;

- Eat fresh, whole foods in their natural state as often as possible; they're high in disease-fighting antioxidants, phytochemicals, and fiber;

Food Recommendations

To improve quality, energy, enzyme content, and pH in a healthy diet, please consider the following recommendations.

Superior Energy-Enhancing Foods

Legumes
Garbanzo beans
Great Northern beans
Kidney beans
Lentils
Lima beans
Mungbean sprouts
Soybean
Soybean curd (tofu)
Soybean sprouts
Split peas
Sunflower sprouts

Vegetables
Artichokes
Broccoli
Brussels sprouts
Cabbage
Cauliflower
Celery
Chinese cabbage
Cucumbers
Dandelion greens
Eggplant

Escarole
Green beans
Green peas
Green pepper
Kale
Mushrooms
Okra
Olives
Onions
Parsley
Spinach
Tomatoes
Watercress
Zucchini

Grains
Barley
Bulgar wheat
Millet
Oatmeal (steel cut)
Rice bran
Rye berries (cracked)
Wheat berries (red)
Wheat germ (raw)
Whole rye bread
 (no wheat)

Whole rye crackers
Wild rice

Nuts and seeds
Almonds (raw)
Cashews (raw)
Macadamia nuts
Peanuts
Pine nuts (raw)
Pumpkin seeds (raw)
Sesame seeds (raw)
Sunflower seeds (raw)

Fruits
Apples
Avocado
Grapefruit
Grapes
Lemons
Peaches
Pears

Dairy
Homemade kefir
Raw, unpasteurized
 goat cheese

Moderate Energy-Enhancing Foods

Moderate enhancement of energy activity only occurs if your dietary intake of these foods is less than 25 percent at each meal.

Acorn squash

Beets

Brown rice

Butternut squash

Carrots

Cereals

Chicken

Cod (Icelandic)

Corn (grits)

Cottage cheese

Fish

Granola

Haddock (Icelandic)

Lean meats

Mackerel

Mozzarella, skim

Pasta

Ricotta cheese

Rye bread

Salmon (Norwegian)

Tuna, canned in water

Turkey

Veal

White potatoes

Whole-grain breads

Yams and sweet potatoes

Foods to Avoid

The following are energy-depleting, high-stress foods. Avoiding or decreasing your intake of these foods will contribute to a longer health span and keep your QEF balanced.

Additives

Alcohol

Bacon/pork products

Butter

Caffeine

Cream cheese/hard cheese

Drugs

Eggs

GMO foods

Hydrogenated fats (margarine)

Irradiated foods

Mayonnaise

Microwaved foods

Processed and refined oils and foods

Salt (table)

Sodium nitrite meat products

Sour cream

Starches (white flours)

Sugar-containing foods and beverages

Sugars (refined)

- Make fruits, vegetables, whole grains, and legumes your main meal. Let fish, fowl, or lean meats serve as condiments. While most American diets are just the reverse of this recommendation, we make it, nevertheless, knowing that it will enhance your health, improve your QEF, and actually heal many organic problems;

- Eat healthy fats. Not all fats are created equal. Some influence your QEF positively, others negatively. As you will recall, EFAs are the building blocks to eicosanoid hormones. Since we can't synthesize them in our bodies, EFAs *must* be gotten from the food we eat. The most important, *linoleic acid,* is abundant in raw almonds, tofu, avocados, cashews, garbanzo beans, olive oil, sunflower seeds, pumpkin seeds, and other familiar foods. Make sure some of these foods are in your daily diet.

Cold-pressed, extra virgin olive oil, sunflower seeds, macadamia nuts, almonds, and cashews are also excellent sources of other energy-enhancing fats. Unlike animal fats, these fats do not raise blood cholesterol or cause you to gain weight. Most important, make it an ongoing habit to consume saturated fat in the form of raw, unheated coconut butter on a daily basis;

- Avoid American sugars that are processed with 2,4,5-T, a dioxin derivative that is one of the most toxic chemicals known;

- Avoid irradiated food altogether;

- Avoid genetically modified (GMO) foods;

- Drink at least six glasses daily of purified, energized, and hydrated water.

Studies have shown that 35 to 80 percent of cancers can be accounted for by diet. The progressive depletion of health-protecting antioxidants our food once naturally contained has been documented to have increased our risk today of cancer and degenerative disease. Scientific data supporting cancer risk reduction with the introduction of antioxidants into the diet have been documented extensively. With antioxidant levels in our standard American diet too low to protect the body from the increasing levels of chemical carcinogens in the environment, statistics show that, since 1970, we have seen a dramatic rise in the incidence of cancer and other chronic degenerative diseases in the United States.

Back in 1986, television journalist Tom Brokaw reported that even then, there were no sources of uncontaminated drinking water left in the United States This means that even crops that would otherwise be considered "organically grown" were contaminated by the water used to grow them. The widespread demineralization of our soil, the declining nutritional (enzymes) values of our food supply, and the resulting weakening of our bodies' immune systems have all been documented. Indeed, not only is the overwhelming majority of American food depleted of vital antioxidants, enzymes, trace minerals, and phytochemicals, but it also contains carcinogenic chemicals that contribute to carcinogenesis. To obtain 100 percent contaminant-free foods, it is necessary to go outside the United States where food products are grown in rich, unspoiled soil and hydrated with pure water.

Quantum Foods (QFs) are what I call "beyond organic" foods. These foods are grown on nutrient-rich and chemical-free soil in a clean environment. QFs provide the body with a synergistic array of thousands of both common and little-known antioxidants, nutrients, and powerful phytochemical compounds that protect the body's optimal health against the ill effects of today's high levels of pollution and stress. They are rated *Grade 10,* meaning that they radiate biophoton energies superior to those of organic foods, especially when they are blended in specific combinations. (In order to be rated Grade 10, every detail of making a Quantum Food blend, from the planting, gathering, and harvesting to the testing and preparation, is meticulously supervised to ensure complete freshness, purity, potency, and vitality.)

Hundreds of plants and whole foods have been studied to find specific blends that catalyze the body's innate healing and QEF reorganization. These unique Quantum Food formulations weave our QEFs into a synchronous, coherent, and cohesive whole. By reshaping faulty energy patterns, we allow the body to be brought into greater and greater synchrony with itself.

Stanford University's William A. Tiller, Ph.D., and many other leading scientists have documented that there is an energy field surrounding all plants. In photographs (see Figure 10.1 on page 96) made with a Kirlian camera, it is possible to actually see patterns of energy normally invisible to the naked human eye. Notice the luminous pattern of light in the Quantum Food sample (whole food supplement) as compared with an ordinary multivitamin.

Boosting Your Body's Reserves

When we are in our twenties, most of our organs have a high functional capacity or energetic reserve, and our QEF is still strong and resilient in response to stress. This means that the body has the potential to do more than is usually necessary to ward off the negative effects of stress. However, as the body ages, the number of its healthy cells is reduced. The loss of cells means there is less of an organized system to counteract stress, less energetic reserve to fuel repair and regeneration. Hormones are thrown out of balance and nutrients are depleted faster than diet can replenish them.

Imagine a fortress under siege from barbarians. They attack the north wall, killing numerous defenders. So half of those who were posted at the east and west walls come running to the north. Now those walls are left vulnerable, and the barbarians can easily take the fortress from either side! After repeated battles, the body experiences just this phenomenon. Calling in reinforcements from nearby locales leaves those other parts weakened to the point where the ability

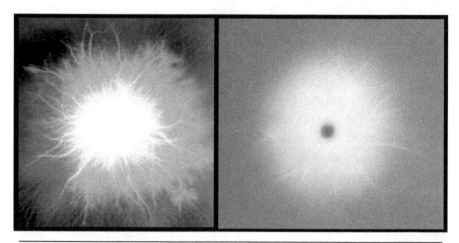

FIGURE 10.1. Kirlian photos of a Quantum Food (left) versus a conventional multivitamin.

to respond adequately to stress and to regain a balanced state of functioning are simply lost. By the time we reach a point where symptoms appear, the process of degeneration is already underway.

Like barbarians, an incessant assault of pollutants taxes the body's adaptive defense mechanisms and diminish the QEF. However, with ample nourishment, the fortress defenders, that is, the hormones and nervous stimuli that help us defend against stress, can ward off insults for decades, possibly a lifetime, without showing many signs of disease. We can better cope with the ever-increasing demands of today's stressful life if we strengthen the body's QEF against stress with Quantum Foods.

We can illustrate the point by relating to you the story of Alfred, who, like many of us, had a problem with cholesterol in his system.

Alfred Challenges Cholesterol

Alfred's maternal grandfather, his mother, and six of his brothers and sisters all suffered from a medical condition called *hypercholesterolemia,* a genetic trait predisposing the individual to build up large amounts of cholesterol in the arteries of the body. An athlete who ran five miles a day, lifted weights, played high school sports, and thought himself to be in top condition, Alfred was surprised to be diagnosed with high cholesterol at the age of twenty-eight. Despite several kinds of prescribed medications, Alfred found himself, at the age of thirty-five, to have the arteries of an obese, sedentary seventy-five-year old man.

One day, his physician ordered a stress test. However, because of the extreme chest pain from an 80-percent blockage of his heart valves with deposited cholesterol, Alfred's cardiac stress test had to be halted. He couldn't even walk up a flight of stairs without gasping for air. Despite treatment with drugs, his condition slowly deteriorated. Apparently out of options, he spent sixteen to twenty hours a day in bed resting. The slightest exertion left him exhausted.

Finally, Alfred consulted a doctor certified in Quantum Medicine. After a comprehensive battery of tests, it was determined that Alfred had extreme liver toxicity and a bone infection in the site where one his wisdom teeth had been extracted ten years ago. A laser dentist removed the infection that was found deep in the bone, and after supplementation with Quantum Foods and following the diet plan outlined in this book, Alfred made a full recovery. His cholesterol count dropped to an acceptable level, and for the first time in years, he was able to resume vigorous physical activity. Recently, Alfred told his doctor, "I just returned from skiing at an altitude of 14,000 feet, and I didn't get out of breath once! I feel like a young athlete again!"

By reducing accumulations of toxins and implementing proper nourishment, Alfred's faulty genetic mechanisms that had programmed him to die of hypercholesterolemia were restored and rebalanced.

Even after it has been abused, the body, with help, has the remarkable ability to cleanse itself of accumulated fats, infections, and toxins and to heal itself.

The Vital Difference of Quantum Foods

Quantum Foods represent blends of the most nutritious food sources on the planet. The nutritional superiority of these foods far exceeds combinations of supplements and even natural, whole foods. A QF supplement must meet extremely high standards of quantum quality:

- **Grade 10, beyond organic.** Growing locations and harvesting methods can cause a plant's mineral content to vary by more than 900 percent. When mineral levels decline, enzyme levels in plants also diminish, in turn causing diminished biophoton levels. This is because an enzyme is a large, energy-radiating protein molecule that contains trace minerals such as zinc, selenium, manganese, and copper. Mineral deficiencies and imbalances that occur when plants are grown in polluted areas with contaminated water contribute to enzyme and biophoton deficiencies. Quantum Foods, on the other hand, contain whole food powders and organ-specific phytonutrients and phytochemicals derived from the deep central forests in India, the wilds of South American rainforests, and the pristine mountaintops of China. The response to Quantum Foods in the meridians of thousands of patients has shown that QFs are perfectly balanced.

- **Toxin-free and biologically active.** Believe it or not, up to 97.5 percent of so-called natural food supplements are either toxic or ineffective. Routine herbal contamination occurs because many product manufacturers accept the Certificate of Analysis from their suppliers, which only requires the testing of harmful bacteria and mold. Rarely are these products tested for toxic contaminants. A high percentage of supplements contain synthetic, isolated vitamins and/or inorganic minerals that deplete enzymes by stimulating rather than by balancing and supporting weak physiology. Many also contain toxic binders, fillers, and flowing agents, such as the suspected carcinogen talcum powder.

    Distinctly different, QFs provide highly bioactive ingredients that are fresh and grown in ideal locations. In addition, they are not irradiated, fumigated, or contaminated with pesticide and/or insecticide residues. They are meticulously tested and retested to be free of common supplemental toxins such as polyvinylpyrrolidone, magnesium stearate, waxes, and many other known or suspected carcinogens.

    To prevent exposure to routine fumigation at ports of passage en route to the United States, QFs are packaged in protective drums with tamper-proof locking pins. Moreover, QFs are prepared with no heat, high pressure, or toxic glues that are commonly used by tablet manufacturers.

- **Organ/tissue specificity.** Phytochemicals are absorbed by the body in a process of selective uptake. Years of extensive clinical research have gone into designing QFs to target and strengthen specific organs or glands of the body without the risk of infectious prion exposure—characteristic of mad cow disease. To further minimize prion risks, QFs are packaged in vegetable capsules, thus eliminating the need for the common preservative used in gelatin capsules.

- **Balanced and balancing.** Taking synthetic supplements, such as vitamins, herbs, hormones, or eating foods that over-stimulate certain hormones has a tendency to unbalance the body, forcing our adrenals into an Alarm Reaction. Our immune system is then stimulated beyond its normal balance, and many facets of immune cell defense are blocked. With Quantum Foods, however, the balanced herbal nutrients simultaneously raise and balance the levels of white blood cells within normal limits.

Digestive Enzymes

Hundreds of reactions that support our antioxidant defense process are regulated by enzymes. In the healthy body, enzyme interaction is harmonized and synchronized. When enzymes are out of sync, or when there are simply too few of them, the body cannot use vitamins and minerals to produce adequate amounts of energy. Quantum Foods (QFs) contain high amounts of enzymes to address this problem. The benefit of these food-based enzymes to cells is vastly superior to many common digestive enzymes available in today's market.

QFs bypass weak intestinal functions while simultaneously strengthening the digestive system. Digestion, the process of breaking down foods into simpler components so that nutrients may be absorbed and assimilated in the digestive tract, involves a maze of biochemical enzyme reactions. Each reaction is dependent upon many cofactors and complex forms of nutrients, as they are found in whole foods of superior quality. Through this process, nutrients reach the cells.

However, in an Alarm Reaction, blood is diverted away from the digestive tract, reducing digestive function dramatically. Supporting the digestive system with fungal-free digestive enzymes may prove beneficial. Remember, enzymes are pH sensitive, and they are blocked by eating too many acid-promoting foods (animal proteins) or by consuming excessive amounts of processed, enzyme-dead, or cooked foods.

Quantum Foods are effective as front line intervention in some of the most difficult health puzzles, and Gina's story was a most challenging puzzle! Let me tell you her story.

Gina Confronts Irritable Bowel Syndrome

As Gina turned forty years of age, she felt depressed and pessimistic about her future. For years, she had been struggling with low energy, insomnia, anxiety, shoulder and neck pain, allergies, and a weak immune system. Her many doctors had not been able to unravel the mystery of her progressive sickness. After years of searching for a doctor who could tell her what was wrong with her, Gina found a physician who diagnosed irritable bowel syndrome (IBS). This condition occurs when undigested food irritates the sensitive linings of the digestive tract, and they become porous and inflamed.

Gina was not able to digest foods because her body was too acidic. Therefore, rotting and fermented food passing through her digestive tract resulted in intestinal irritation. Additionally, these undigested food residues had penetrated into her liver, causing an array of debilitating symptoms, including those of premature aging.

While Gina was thankful to finally have a credible diagnosis, she and her doctor still were not sure why her digestive system was not working properly, why she couldn't digest her food completely. She thought her problem might be related to gallbladder surgery she'd had ten years earlier. Her doctor referred her to a nutritionist.

The nutritionist noticed that Gina's digestive system was so inflamed that it would be necessary for her to eliminate the consumption of meats, dairy products, and eggs from her diet, as research had shown that eating less food or easier-to-digest food stopped accelerated aging of the digestive system. A friend referred Gina to a physician certified in Quantum Medicine. After a comprehensive series of tests, he confirmed the diagnosis of the nutritionist—and concurred, to some degree, on the diet recommendations. However, he instituted a regimen of Quantum Foods. Following the diet plan outlined in this book, Gina was restored to full health within a period of less than a year. Now she could follow the "normal" American diet, but she said, "No, I'm sticking to the Quantum Food diet."

Feeding the Body and the QEF

In order to appreciate the importance of high-quality Quantum Foods, it is useful to consider how the food we eat supports the body's functioning. We can start by considering the human body as an electrical system. The electrical wires are the invisible acupuncture meridians and nerve connections that conduct and transmit life-giving energy to all body organs and systems. Before power can be put through a wire, the system must have the correct insulation and resistance in place. Insufficient insulation and resistance can cause an electrical short circuit in the body or blockage of cellular communication systems. For nutrition to be effective beyond the chemical level, the body must be nourished energetically. This neglected area of nutritional science can recapture the state of well being that slips away as we age.

Many functions of the body's organs and glands are dependent upon how efficiently these organs and glands communicate with one another. The human body has a complex, amazingly fast, and powerful communication system.

Communication involves the transfer of information in three ways: electrically, chemically, and electromagnetically. This complex communication network depends on hormones and neurotransmitters that help carry signals along nerve pathways to special cellular receptor sites. As they travel through the body, signal-bearing hormones search out a place to deliver their messages. Receptors, poised to receive these signals on the surface of cells, play a major role in regulating the body, acting in a way similar to the way a radio receiver picks up invisible signals that travel through the air from a transmitter only if the radio is tuned to the correct frequency. At the incorrect frequency, there is no communication. Ah, but at the correct frequency, you do have reception: clear transmission of sound information.

Quantum Foods rejuvenate cellular function by fueling cells with enzymes and mineral catalysts that provide the raw ingredients for the body to nourish itself, physically and energetically. Molecules of the DNA and cellular structures actually vibrate to the subtle energies of enzymes as they radiate a specific vibratory frequency that helps to fine-tune, stabilize, and amplify hormone transmission and reception in the body.

The incredible powers of these nutritional factors are being uncovered in many prestigious laboratories across the world. There is mounting evidence that these awesome vibratory energies can penetrate deep within the molecular biology of a cell to reach the aging control center. Scientists have already identified how these incredible energy-packed nutrients strike at the very heart of the aging process by re-synchronizing the body's energetic communication systems.

When our bodies are functioning normally, billions of our cells simultaneously receive signals from biophotons and hormones and convert their chemicals into electrochemical energy. These electrochemical energies also excite nerve fibers that send neural impulses racing through the brain in vital neural regulation routines. This truly awesome system can fire off signals through the nerves at a rate of one thousand messages a second. But fueling all this complexity, the basic building block of the nervous system, the brain, the spinal cord, and other nerves, is the neuron itself. The neuron is an amazing miniaturized chemical factory that needs 15 billion atoms of oxygen per second. A reduction in this oxygen supply due to reductions in blood supply can create electrical disturbances in the body. The nervous system begins to radiate disharmonic electrical impulses that interfere with the energetic control centers of the body.

Our cells require a delicate and subtle balance of nutrients that must be maintained by the quality of food we eat. Amino acids, vitamins functioning as coenzymes, and fatty acids all have a direct influence on the electrical stability of the body's cells. In fact, more than 300 nutrient ratios must be in balance for optimal electrochemical communication in the body.

The cellular/nutrient connection is well documented in most authoritative textbooks. However, this information is not studied in any depth by students in medical school. Receiving only preliminary instruction in nutrition and hormone physiology, medical students then generally pursue detailed studies of pharmaceutical drugs, many of which destroy enzymes and cause severe hormone and nutrient imbalances.

There are thousands of enzyme-controlled reactions in the body. Deficits in hormone production and reception are found at specific points where great demands for enzymes exist. Magnesium, for example, is a critical nutrient needed during several stages of the cell's energy cycles. My own research has shown a high correlation between intracellular magnesium deficiency and an acid pH, and deficits in nerve and hormonal transmission. This study, published in the *Journal of Applied Nutrition,* found that many forms of vitamins and minerals do not reach and nourish the cells of the body. I discovered that enzymatic forms of magnesium improve the electrochemical balance of cells while other forms of magnesium had no effect. The reason: the latter were inorganic and lacked enzymes. Thus, sometimes, you might take what you believe to be the correct substance, but it does not produce the desired effect. This is not the case with Quantum Foods.

pH and the GI Tract: The Immunity Connection

"GI" refers to the gastrointestinal tract, your intestines. Research tells us that there is a connection between the GI tract and delayed healing responses. This subtle connection is finally getting some long-overdue attention. For example, at Cornell University, Jeffrey Gates is studying how dietary patterns affect bacteria populations in the GI tract. According to Gates, acid-producing meats provide an ideal environment for the growth of unhealthy pathogenic bacteria. He believes the intestines are a battleground for millions of bacteria. Thus, when the digestive process is weak, unhealthy bacteria can outnumber and kill healthy bacteria, paving the way for many stress-associated diseases. In essence, an imbalance in intestinal bacteria can become an additional stressor to the body's QEF.

Just like soil needs the right pH balance to grow healthy plants, the intestinal flora of your digestive system needs the right pH for food to be broken down into nutrients. Acid-promoting foods and processed foods are generally not fully digested and cause prolonged irritation to the GI tract. These foods acidify the body and block digestive enzyme activity. Food rots, ferments, and putrefies, making the intestines a breeding ground for unhealthy bacteria and yeast and fungal infections.

The economy of the body depends to a large extent on a smoothly functioning GI system. Digestion is the body's most energy-consuming process. To see this at work, recall the case of Gina and her battle with irritable bowel syndrome. Because all her organ's reserves of nutrients were depleted, her body had been attempting to compensate for her GI incompetence by escalating metabolism, thereby depleting reserves of glucose and protein in her liver and tissues. Gina's body was depleted like an overdrawn bank account. For years, her body had used up too much energy, allowing reserves of critical nutrients to cause her pH to drop deeper and deeper into the danger zone of acidity, where enzymes become inactive.

When the body is too acidic and toxic, digestive fluids become irritant and inflammatory, increasing intestinal permeability (leaky gut syndrome) and the absorption of gut-produced toxins (endotoxins). When the intestines are more permeable, the immune cells do not receive adequate nourishment, and the body is no longer protected from toxins and microbes.

Normally, the liver has a special enzyme system to render environmental toxins harmless, causing toxins to be excreted via the urine and eliminated via bile into the intestines. But when the intestinal walls become too inflamed, the absorption and transport of hormone-enhancing nutrients to the liver become blocked. Once the intestinal barrier function is breached, the immune system and liver are overstimulated and overworked.

When enzymes are deficient—or blocked by an acidic pH—toxins are dumped into the bile and stored in the gallbladder. Since these toxins are irritating to the gallbladder, they are often dumped inappropriately and excessively into the small intestines, causing inflammation of the pancreatic duct. Thus, in Gina's case, it was her long-standing pH problem that was the cause of her gallbladder problem, rather than the latter being the root of her chronic illness. Once we dealt with the pH problem, the gallbladder cleared up, and so did her chronic illness. There was no "magic bullet," just a thorough understanding of Gina's body chemistry and its relation to Quantum Foods.

Quantum Foods to Restore Liver and GI Function

The liver's level of functioning and its detoxification ability determine how effective our anti-aging immune defenses will be, in part because all anti-aging hormones pass through the liver before reaching their designated receptor sites. In the early stages of irritable bowel syndrome (IBS), the liver, which also is responsible for preparing and dispersing nutrients into the bloodstream for delivery elsewhere in the body, is working overtime to remove undigested food molecules and to oxidize intestine-produced toxins. Eventually, however, the liver fatigues and becomes functionally weak, and we must deal with the syndrome.

The liver's role in accelerated aging and immune disorders, ignored by most physicians, was critically important in Gina's case, discussed on page 99. As you will recall, she was deficient in many different hormones. In order to restore normal functioning to her digestive system, Gina needed to be on a highly specialized diet of bioactive peptides, stabilized rice bran, organic colostrum, and vegetable concentrates to gently enhance detoxification functions. Gina's nutritionist advised her that these whole food concentrates would enhance her QEF and have regenerative effects on her gut and liver.

After three months on this nutritional program, Gina's digestive system improved, and she was able to absorb energy-enhancing nutrients into her cells. As her energy levels improved, so did her immune function and its ability to repair damage in her body.

When the liver is overburdened and overloaded with toxins, many hormones needed elsewhere in the body get trapped there. Even though a person may take a hormone supplement, it may not be able to reach receptor sites in the GI tract or in other organs.

Our clinical research has demonstrated that by consuming nutrient-dense Quantum Foods, it is possible to rest the GI tract without unduly onerous dietary restrictions. When the body digests Quantum Foods, the delicate linings of the GI tract are not irritated or stressed.

QUANTUM FOODS FOR LIFE EXTENSION

When taken together, life-stretching superfoods and superior herbal complexes, all bonded with enzymes and biologically active nutritional factors, penetrate cells at incredible speeds and with amazing efficiency, enhancing natural hormone production and reception. Conversely, taking synthetic hormones and vitamins is like trying to play beautiful music after tuning only a few notes on the piano. There is no comparison to the healing effects of the nutrients found in Quantum Foods (QFs) as they work in harmony to combat stress within the molecular biology of our cells—right where aging begins!

Specifically, QF nutrients synchronize and protect the integrity of cells by snuffing out youth-stealing free radicals that corrupt the genetic material of cells and rob us of healing energy. As the body restores its natural rhythms and harmonic vibrations, our cells function at more youthful levels. And, most important, antistress hormones increase to youthful levels.

Phytonutrient-rich QFs attempt to follow Hippocrates's famous adage, "Let food be thy medicine and medicine be thy food." The use of QFs combined with novel methods of transporting nutrients through carrier and *channel proteins* via high-energy complexes of synergistic ingredients offers a new strategy for boosting nutrient absorption by the cells.

QFs are also rich in phytonutrients. Although vegetables and fruits contain a great variety of phytochemicals that protect against cancer, the quality and quantity of these phytochemicals vary greatly depending upon agricultural practices, water and air pollution levels, and soil ecology. Decades of reckless and unconscionable handling of chemical toxins have contributed to widespread water, air, and food pollution. The increase in cancer due to suspected and known carcinogens has turned into a demand from the public to have chemicals tested and retested for human safety before they reach consumers and for cleaner, more potent food supplements. However, with QFs, we have no such concerns.

"So," you ask, "what are these Quantum Foods you keep talking about?"

I'm glad you asked. In the next section, we will recommend the best of them.

THE TOP TWELVE QUANTUM FOODS

In the war against cancer and other stress-associated disorders, scientists have identified certain foods that are among the richest sources of active nutrients. These sources provide nourishment that is hundreds, or maybe even thousands, of times greater than conventional foods and far surpass common nutritional supplements.

Following are the top twelve of the most powerful and highest quality QF ingredients—the most nutritionally dense foods on the planet. These are not just high-quality foods available in local health food stores, but specially harvested and formulated Quantum Foods.

1. Young Barley Grass

For superior QEF enhancement, we only recommend non-GMO (genetically modified) and non-hybrid green barley grass from South America. This amazing whole food has 200 times more magnesium and 8,000 times more potassium than a similar serving of most vegetables. With 45 percent protein and thousands of different enzymes, this Quantum Food has a wide spectrum of nature's finest ingredients. Warning: juicing young barley and/or compressing it into a tablet destroys its radiant energy.

2. Stabilized Rice Bran and Protein

This is a storehouse of precious but delicate nutrients called *tocotrienols.* These super nutrients have 6,000 times greater antioxidant activity than vitamin E. Destroyed by cooking and common processing and preparation methods in the nutritional industry, this stabilized rice bran does not oxidize and is easy to digest and assimilate. This Quantum Food has more than 100 powerful antioxidants that are preserved using a newly developed proprietary technology to protect and preserve their fragile molecular structures. In addition, this Quantum Food provides *gamma oryzanol,* a cholesterol antioxidant, *ferulic acid,* a cancer antioxidant, and *alpha lipoic acid,* the body's universal antioxidant that can improve your metabolism, stabilize your blood sugar, limit sugar cravings, and regenerate the levels of other antioxidants to provide a spectacular boost for the immune system.

3. Bioactive Peptides

Bioactive peptides are biologically active protein complexes, not to be compared to amino acids (traditionally defined as the building blocks of protein). This unique form of protein extracted from the whey of milk and naturally available in blue-green algae helps to improve peptide hormone production while maintaining balance between insulin and glucagon, and between insulin and HGH—a proteinlike hormone secreted naturally by the pituitary gland. Care must be taken to ensure that whey peptides (polypeptides, dipeptides, and tripeptides) be air dried and not heat damaged, as most whey products are loaded with harmful byproducts like MSG and mutilated proteins that cause DNA instability. However, when combined with high-energy carbohydrate compounds from rice syrup solids, these peptides promote the rapid absorption of protein into the cells, thereby enhancing quantum coherence and the full strength of the QEF. Peptides contain neural and hormonal-regulating factors that help to maintain all functions of the body on an even keel, neither overactive nor underactive. Combining peptides with conjugated linoleic acid (CLA)—a fatty acid that possesses a unique and potent antioxidant activity as well as anticancer properties—stabilizes DNA and prevents genetic mutations.

4. Japanese Spirulina

Spirulina that comes from the pristine mountainous areas of Japan is far superior to other spirulina sources. It is exceptionally rich in nutrients, contains 70 percent protein of the highest quality, and is free of pesticides and other chemicals.

5. Coconut Butter

As mentioned earlier, coconut butter must be unheated, raw, free of harmful solvents, and not deodorized, bleached, or hydrogenated, as are most commercially available sources. When in this state, coconut butter is a rich source of the MCFAs (medium chain fatty acids) that maintain the stability of biophotons and clear out harmful trans-fatty acids from cellular structures. QF coconut butter always means *non-hydrogenated* coconut butter. Avoid the hydrogenated form, which diminishes the QEF and clogs cells with fats; the organic coconut butters are hydrogenated, even though the label doesn't indicate hydrogenation.

6. Pollen

Pollen is a high-energy Quantum Food that is 100 percent allergen-free and pesticide-free. Unlike many pollen sources, Quantum pollen is not exposed to heat, moisture, sunlight, air, chemical treatment, and harmful gas, which are used to sterilize ordinary pollens. Quantum medical practitioners use a multiple pollen extract that has a broader range of benefits than any single pollen extract. Harvested from healthy bees from a super-clean environment, this product is alive with enzymes, has a broad spectrum of nutrients, and contains more than 38 percent pure protein. While most pollen spoils quickly even when refrigerated, we found that when this incredible Quantum Food is combined with stabilized rice bran, it is possible to maintain its freshness and continued viability over time.

7. Fungal-Free Digestive Enzymes

Specially formulated, fungal-free enzymes are the first digestive enzymes without fungal residues; they are completely free of animal-source enzymes associated with "mad cow disease." We use a full spectrum of plant enzymes to support the digestion of fat, protein, starch, lactose, sugar, and fiber. The unmatched enzymatic activity of this combination, along with rich organic acids and substrates, enhances the body's own ability to produce digestive enzymes.

8. Propolis

A natural antibiotic resin produced by bees, propolis is extremely hard to find. Recently, I found propolis that was free of arsenic, silicon dioxide, and pesticides. It has a short shelf life and is commonly found spoiled and loaded with pesticides. Now, however, you can experience the powerful anti-infective, antioxidant, and healing properties of this unique Quantum Food without any toxic chemicals or harmful processing methods. As a bonus, researchers have documented that propolis has powerful anticancer properties.

9. Royal Jelly

A superfood that bees produce to feed the queen bee, royal jelly from South America is the best source of B vitamins that help fuel energy cycles. Vitamin B_{12} is probably the single most important nutrient depleted by stress. Essential for proper mental functioning, vitamin B_{12} is not absorbed when the body pH drops and the stomach fails to produce hydrochloric acid, pepsin, and intrinsic factor—a factor necessary for absorption. The crystalline forms of vitamin B_{12} deplete enzymes and may block hormone activity. Nature provides us with superior B vitamins in South American royal jelly that can rapidly assimilate into our cells.

10. Organic Colostrum

A special fluid secreted by a mother several days after birth to give highly protective, immune-boosting factors to her offspring, organic colostrum is rich in MSM, a natural sulfur compound used for treating inflammation disorders. Organic colostrum is also rich in human-active immunoglobulins (IgG, IgM, IgA) and lactoferrin to help boost immunity. Unlike defatted commercial colostrum with its toxic antibiotic and chemical residues, 100 percent whole and organic colostrum (from cows) has been found to qualify as a Quantum Food.

11. Adaptogenic Herbs

My research described in Chapter 1 led me to experiment with blends of destressing roots and herbs (Indian Somalata, Siberian Maral Root, Arctic Root, Tibetan Ginseng, Fo-Ti). In the twenty-first century, we need some broad-based support to help our bodies cope with the heavy demands and stresses of modern life, and the QEF-organizing patterns of these rare and precious herbal combinations provide the body with quantum nourishment that is far beyond any one of them alone.

12. Immune-Boosting Herbs

In my search to uncover plants that would repair my damaged adrenals and kidneys, I came across those that augmented my body's immune system battles against viruses and infections. Clinical trials with these herbal combinations made the critical difference in my own case, as well as those of thousands of patients assessed with a variety of immune deficiencies.

I have merged ancient food wisdom with the latest science to find the most important QFs available in the world. Remember, unlike conventional nutrition, the above QFs work in concert with your body's healing dimension. Moreover, researchers are continuing to discover new compounds in these foods that may have even greater health benefits.

Quantum foods, made up of critical nutrients and phytochemicals, inhibit overstimulation of the adrenals and pancreas, and enhance hormones depleted by the Alarm Reaction. As we will discuss in the next chapter, the Quantum Energy Diet is not about counting calories or avoiding fats and cholesterol. It simply prescribes *more* energy-enhancing foods that *enhance* the body's natural balance of hormones, and *fewer* energy-depleting foods that *upset* that natural balance. This is not an ultra-limited, boring diet plan. Once you understand which foods provoke the Alarm Reaction, you will be able to eat an endless variety of foods that will invoke a healthy response.

The healing of our bodies is a gift of immeasurable worth. The quality of our foods directly affects the amount of energy in reserve that we have for unexpected life or health crises.

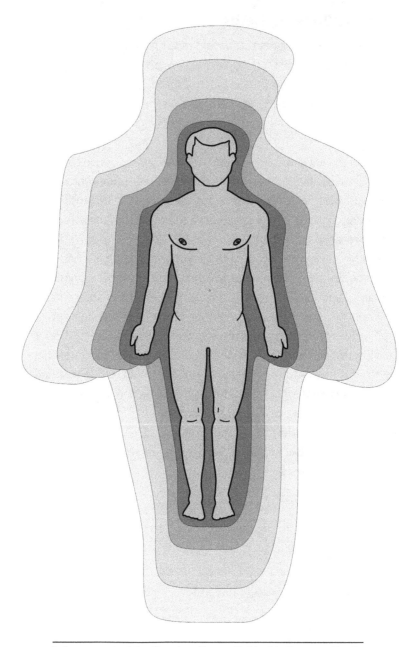

Enhancement of the Quantum Energy Field with Quantum Foods.

11

The Quantum
Energy Diet

In this age of diet fads and fast foods, the best eating plan may be the oldest. In Biblical times, people lived on whole grains, fruits, nuts, greens, legumes, and olive oil, only consuming small amounts of animal protein. Their diet was filled with fiber, lean protein, antioxidants, phytochemicals, and phytonutrients, and was low in fat, sodium, and cholesterol.

A diet that contains plenty of phytochemicals can help prevent heart disease and cancer, reduce blood pressure, and slow the effects of aging. These naturally occurring compounds lay an antioxidant-rich foundation that's inhospitable to toxins, free radicals, and other stressors. Moreover, they help to *eliminate* free radicals that damage our DNA, the source of healing and intelligence in the body.

Can eating vegetables promote healing and prolong your life? Many mainstream scientists think so. Experts are now convinced that the right dietary choices can extend life span and keep us younger, healthier, and stronger as we go through life.

Since 1983, the plant-based, almost meatless diets of Asia have been studied by a team of researchers working with the China-Cornell-Oxford Diet and Health Projects. One of the project researcher, Dr. T. C. Campbell, reported that a mostly vegan diet results in a significant reduction in many age-associated diseases.

AVOID FOODS THAT INCREASE STRESS OR PROVOKE THE ALARM REACTION

Certain foods and additives—organic compounds in foods—block or lessen the body's production of specific useful hormones. Caffeine, sugars, refined flours, and simple starches overload the endocrine system by throwing hormones out of balance and triggering the Alarm Reaction. Remember, every time we allow foods to trigger an Alarm Reaction, our stress levels increase dramatically. And, when our stress levels rise, our QEF decreases and overall health is diminished.

Foods that contain caffeine or related compounds block the production of DHEA and natural progesterone.

High intake of saturated fat diminishes hormone levels in many individuals, especially the trans-fatty acids, which have the added effect of blocking or inhibiting biophoton flow and communication with the acupuncture meridian system.

Consuming too many acid-forming foods *decreases* the body's production of hormones and biophotons and suppresses immunity, while long-term ingestion of alkaline-promoting foods *increases* hormone and biophoton activity. Ideally, the pH (acid and alkaline balance) of the food we eat should be compatible with the body's pH: 75 percent alkaline and 25 percent acid. However, most diets, even vegetarian diets, are the opposite: 75 percent acid and 25 percent alkaline. Most people are surprised that even a vegetarian diet can be so acidic because we tend to think of animal-based proteins as the primary culprits of over-acidity in the body. But because all grains are also acid-producing, vegetarians can be just as susceptible to an overly acidic diet as those who consume meats. On the other hand, citrus fruits, which many would assume to be highly acidic are actually extremely alkaline. Reactions that people commonly have to these fruits occur not because the fruit is acidic, but because the individual is acidic! It is the clash of opposite ends of the pH spectrum—alkaline citrus fruit to acid body—that creates the familiar internal upsets.

The excess acidity in the "typical" American diet depletes alkaline minerals and blocks enzymes that are involved in converting phytochemicals into hormones, or that are involved in removing harmful substances from our bodies. In addition, when our pH drops into the acid zone, the functional efficiency of our organs and glands also drops. This often results in a lack of stomach hydrochloric acid, and bile that is acidic, rather than alkaline. When bile is acidic, we don't break down fats into EFAs and eicosanoid hormones (prostaglandins). In addition, the acid bile (which research by physiologists has shown to be optimal only at an alkaline 8.0 pH) inactivates all pancreatic enzymes. Inactivation of these enzymes results in poor assimilation of nutrients and a high infiltration of toxins into the blood and lymph systems as undigested food passes through the intestinal tract.

During the first few months on the Quantum Energy Diet, it may be necessary to energize the digestive system with fresh herbs such as ginger, peppermint, and fresh ground fennel and caraway seeds or take fungal-free digestive enzymes (see the Resources section for information). Adding these herbs to your daily Quantum Energy Diet will help you digest and assimilate nutrients more efficiently.

How Much Protein?

Myths abound regarding how much protein we need to stay healthy. For years experts have told us that a diet that is 30 percent protein is ideal; the animal food-products industry says it's closer to 36 percent.

Perhaps we may find a clue as to our protein requirements by looking at human mother's milk. When we were babies, our bodies were growing faster than they would ever grow again, doubling birth weight in only six months. Yet, those of us who were breast-fed received only 2.5 to 3 percent protein in our diet!

For a long time, nutrition experts believed that animal protein was superior to plant protein. Grains, legumes, nuts, seeds, vegetables, tubers, and fruits were acknowledged as containing vital nutrients and fiber while their protein content was generally portrayed as a poor substitute for meat or milk.

According to researchers such as Dr. T. C. Campbell, Professor of Biochemistry at Cornell University, among others, current intakes of meat and dairy products are a major cause of our high rates of cancer, heart disease, diabetes, obesity, and osteoporosis. His long-term research into the diets of other cultures has revealed that a diet lower in animal protein and higher in plant protein results in a longer health span. A vegetarian diet provides adequate protein, fiber, and nutrients, and has the added advantage of balancing the body's pH.

Researchers working with the China-Cornell-Oxford Diet and Health Projects report that all the protein we need can be provided by a vegetarian diet, with the added advantage of reducing the risk of many age-associated diseases.

In fact, most vegetables have far more than the 3 percent of protein that we saw in the breast-fed infant's diet. All the protein that we need to make hormones and keep insulin balanced can easily be had without eating meat. Plant-based foods are loaded with biologically active forms of protein bound to minerals and enzymes. And, when we eat plant foods, we assimilate more of the available protein without an expenditure or depletion of energy in the digestive tract. Further, plant proteins do not produce sufficient acids to stress our buffering systems.

Conversely, however, consuming excessive animal protein overstimulates

Proteins Found in Plants

We do not need to eat a diet rich in meat and dairy products to get sufficient protein in a healthy diet. Proteins are found in abundance in many
common plant foods:

Plant Food	Protein
spinach	49 percent
broccoli	45 percent
lettuce	34 percent
soybeans	43 percent
lentils	29 percent
wheat germ	31 percent
pumpkin seeds	29 percent
sunflower seeds	23 percent
oatmeal	14 percent

the body's buffering or acid-neutralizing system. In order to decrease this acidity, the body will draw alkaline ash minerals from the tissue and organs of the
body. Over time, this process depletes the body's reserves of energy, and then its
very substance, wasting muscle and bone.

Saturated Fats and Trans-Fats

The two primary dietary mistakes made in this country are either consuming
too much saturated fat or, at the other extreme, maintaining a diet devoid of
fats. Levels of fat intake directly effect energy flow, hormone activity and production, and a host of other functions in the body.

Despite the common belief that all fats are bad, we should *not* avoid all fats!
Without fats, the body's billions of cells cannot regulate the transport of nutrients and hormones, and your QEF will become weakened. Without fats, hormones cannot form or function, nor can cells function properly. Our bodies
need a steady supply of dietary fats from olive oil, coconut oil, nuts, seeds,
olives, and avocados. In addition, our research has shown that hormone production also can be enhanced when we consume adequate amounts of oils
found in cold-water fish like salmon and mackerel.

Meats, cheese, eggs, and milk are high in unhealthy saturated fats. Restricting saturated fat while consuming plant-based fats combined with biologically active proteins is the best long-range approach to enhancing natural hormone production. For most people, this means cutting down greatly on consumption of red meats, eggs, and dairy products such as milk, cheese, and butter.

When oils are processed and heated at high temperatures, they contain *trans-fats.* You can identify trans-fats in foods by looking for the words "hydrogenated" or "partially hydrogenated" in the ingredients list. Many breads, baked goods, chocolate, frozen dinners, and processed meat products contain hydrogenated fats. Trans-fats block hormone production and activity and clog the circulatory system. The consequences of eating too much of these animal-derived saturated fats include high blood pressure (potentially leading to stroke), high blood cholesterol, adult-onset diabetes, and arthritis. Eating too much of the wrong fats may also contribute to the development of cancer and heart disease. If you want longevity and vibrant health, don't eat them.

Both animal-derived saturated fats and trans-fats block the balanced productions of *eicosanoid* hormones. These powerful hormones (prostaglandins, thromboxanes, leukotrienes, and lipoxins), derived from essential fatty acids (EFAs), control the immune system, the nervous system, the heart, the reproductive system, and the endocrine system. There are both good and bad eicosanoids. The good eicosanoids are powerful, fast-acting hormones that control the production of other hormones throughout the body. Dependent on pH control mechanisms, these hormones serve as hormonal-activating and control systems. Bad eicosanoids produce pain and inflammation and weaken the immune system. When bad eicosanoids are elevated above good eicosanoids, hormone activity and production drops dramatically. When the body has more "good" and fewer "bad" eicosanoids, hormone production and activity increases and the body's QEF is enhanced.

THE QUANTUM ENERGY DIET

The Quantum Energy Diet differs from other diet plans in that it merges ancient food wisdom and the latest science to activate and nourish your QEF. Beyond drugs, vitamin supplements, or any single herb, nothing even comes close to the life-giving power of whole foods.

The foods emphasized in this diet plan work in harmony with your meridian energies to restore balance on many levels. And, as you have read in previous chapters, these goals are specifically to:

• Provide phytochemical-rich foods with proven health benefits, including the prevention of cancer, heart disease, and arthritis, and the correction of hormone-related disorders.

- Stabilize your pH and detoxification functions, so you can healthfully neutralize and excrete toxins from your body regularly.

- Stabilize your DNA by protecting your body with plant-based antioxidants that can neutralize free radicals. Stabilizing DNA also has the added effect of boosting your biophoton levels, which prevents stress from overwhelming you or doing damage to your body.

- Stabilize your hormonal balance and heart-brain resonance with foods that enhance hormone and neurotransmitter communication.

- Improve immunity with foods that maximize your immune response or that have natural antiviral or anti-infective properties.

- Evoke your inner powers of healing by increasing the penetration and flow of light energies or biophotons.

The Quantum Energy Diet emphasizes foods that contain natural plant-based hormones and hormone-stimulating phytochemicals. For example, foods made from the soybeans—including tofu, tempeh, and roasted soybeans—contain isoflavones, a naturally occurring form of estrogen. Eaten daily, these foods can help prevent hot flashes, night sweats, and other symptoms related to estrogen deficiency. Whole oats, corn, basmati rice, raw ginger, and fresh tomatoes are melatonin-rich foods and help to restore heart-brain resonance. Coconut oil, yams, and carrots contain small amounts of DHEA precursors and help to stimulate natural DHEA production.

When followed consistently, along with a daily program of exercise, the Quantum Energy Diet will enhance the body's ability to manufacture hormones and biophotons, as well as enhance and strengthen the immune system.

In cultures such as the Pakistani Hunzukuts, the Yucatans, the Chihuahua Indians, and the Abkhazians of Russia, similar diets have resulted in extremely low incidences of cancer, heart disease, ear disorders, and many of the other illnesses endemic to the American lifestyle.

Extensive research has shown that Quantum Energy Foods can do the following:

- Replenish the cellular levels of enzyme-bound minerals (magnesium, potassium, calcium, and sodium);

- Reduce the depletion of DHEA and hundreds of other hormones;

- Improve fatty acid metabolism and levels of fatty acids critical to hormone production and circulatory health of the body;

- Maximize energy metabolism in all the cells of the body;

- Reduce the intake of chemical toxins that aggravate symptoms and block hormone production;

- Excrete these toxins gradually, allowing the body to stay energetic and healthy. Although it is necessary and critical that these toxins be eliminated, releasing them too quickly can dangerously deplete energy and cause an endless array of symptoms. The Quantum Energy Diet helps to release these toxins slowly.

Since digestion is the body's most energy-consuming process, this diet program is designed to conserve energy needed for rejuvenation and detoxification. The process of rejuvenation requires a steady and consistent level of energy provided by foods that are whole and fresh, and high in water content, phytochemicals, biologically active protein, and alkalinity.

Packed with phytochemicals and antioxidants, the Quantum Energy Diet provides superior nourishment and the *optimal* balance of protein, carbohydrates, and fats. Most important, this diet plan is designed to enhance the dynamics of your QEF.

Stress, emotional as well as dietary, lowers pH and depletes protein. Under stress, the body can resort to the inappropriate cannibalistic utilization of protein. This diet plan *maintains* pH so that the body can digest, absorb, and assimilate protein efficiently. A high intake of animal protein, as advocated by the standard American diet, pyramid diets, and other popular diet plans, causes a progressive acidification of the body's cells. The more acidic we become, the more we *decrease* digestive capacity and *impede* the assimilation of nutrients into our cells. When protein and nutrients are in short supply, the body leaches nutrients from itself, depleting healing energies and accelerating the aging process. The Superior Energy-Enhancing Foods emphasized in the Quantum Energy Diet contain concentrations of protein that *regulate* protein and hormone metabolism, keeping the body's fund of protein safe from being leached by needless stress.

Unlike the popular Zone diet and high-protein diet plans, this *hormone-enhancing* diet accomplishes the following:

- It maintains pH, keeping our pH within optimal limits. Digestion, absorption, assimilation, and the utilization of nutrients improve as pH is brought into the normal range.

- It maintains a healthy pattern of detoxification in the body. When pH is optimal, many enzymes involved in the detoxification of environmental pollutants are able to excrete, rather than store toxins.

- It maintains HDL and LDL cholesterol at optimal levels while fortifying cell membranes against attack by free radicals.

- It maintains the balance between "good" and "bad" eicosanoids.

- It maintains the body's equilibrium between the physical and energetic systems of the body.

- It is designed to maintain and balance the body's immune system, resulting in optimal patterns of regeneration and a longer health span.

- It gives us Mother Nature's own perfect balance of protein, fats, and carbohydrates in the Superior Energy-Enhancing Food Group—provided, of course, that these foods are not GMO, and have not been irradiated. No calorie counting or computations are necessary!

KEEP A DIET DIARY

People who follow this diet typically report more energy, sleep more soundly, and notice that their fingernails become stronger with a healthy pink color beneath the nail bed. These changes reflect better metabolism and circulation and are indications of better health.

Keep a personal health diary for a month or two. Each day, record what you have consumed, and how you feel, look, and sleep, as well as anything you notice about your energy level, regularity, and disposition. With proper nutrition, cells regenerate and revitalize, but often improvement occurs slowly and subtly. A diary will help you track your progress.

By applying the concepts conveyed in this book, you are on the road to a higher level of health. These concepts can mean the difference between misery and well-being—the difference between a long, happy, and healthy life and an unnecessarily shortened life full of discomfort. It can save you a great deal of money and grief from health problems and medical costs. It can eliminate the sense of hopelessness and helplessness that more often than not accompany age-related disorders.

Optimal healing and optimal health require the willingness to learn how hidden stressors from our environment are harming our bodies, and a willingness to make healthy lifestyle changes. Once you accept responsibility for your health, increased vitality and longevity can be your reality.

Quantum Energy Recipes

A low fat and high complex carbohydrate diet, naturally high in fiber and packed with phytochemicals and phytonutrients, leads to a healthy QEF balance. And showing you how you can establish a diet that results in QEF balance and the maintenance of your body's optimum levels of healing energy has been the purpose of this book. This chapter will offer a series of recipes that will help you to put the Quantum Energy Diet into concrete form, day in and day out. Obviously, feel free to modify my ideas based on family likes and dislikes, and make substitutions based on what is available in your area. On the other hand, ordering ingredients by mail may be your best option.

Try to use fresh produce in all of the recipes in this chapter. Fresh produce is vitamin-packed, enzyme-rich, and loaded with nature's nutritional powerhouses: phytochemicals. Always purchase produce that is pesticide- and antibiotic-free. Vary your salads with chicory, escarole, and endive, as these greens are full of enzyme-activating minerals and phytochemicals and help to promote healthy liver detoxification.

QF INGREDIENTS

Before we suggest some QF recipes, we need to consider the pros and cons of some of the standard ingredients.

Whole Grains

Whole grains should be organic and cooked slowly at low temperatures. The highest levels of phytonutrients and biologically active protein and fats are found in old-fashioned, slow-cooked oatmeal, whole wheat and rye berries, and millet. These grains are cooked in the following manner:

1. Rinse the grain thoroughly in a colander.

2. Soak overnight in a bowl.

3. The next morning, bring about 3–4 parts water to 1 part beans to a boil in a non-aluminum cooking pot.

4. Stir in the grain. Return water to a boil, then cover and simmer over low heat until the water is absorbed.

The oily germ of the whole grain has fifty times the phytochemical activity of ground flour. When grain is crushed to make flour, its oily germ is exposed to air and may become rancid. Moisture can cause grains to become stale and/or moldy, so keep flour stored in tightly lidded jars in a cool, dry place. Not all grains are created equal, and some kinds of processing will render even the best grains potentially detrimental to our health. When grains are refined for commercial use, the germ and bran are removed, leaving us with the simple starches that trigger abnormal hormonal responses from the pancreas and adrenal glands, depleting our QEF. Here are some recommendations:

Oatmeal

Instant varieties of oatmeal upset our hormonal responses. Old-fashioned, slow-cooked oatmeal is a perfect hormone balancer.

Rice

Instant rice, rice cakes, overcooked rice, brown rice, and rice drinks throw your hormones out of balance. Slow-cooked, white, basmati rice or wild rice, when combined with legumes, enhances your hormone responses.

Pasta

Pasta made from refined white flour disturbs your hormone balance. Use whole-wheat pasta to keep your hormones balanced.

Bread

Most bread triggers the Alarm Reaction. Whole rye or pumpernickel breads are good hormone balancers. However, be aware that many pumpernickel and rye breads have more refined wheat flour than rye and can thus trigger the Alarm Reaction. A good rule of thumb: If rye flour is listed before wheat flour in the ingredients, it means that the bread contains enough rye flour to keep your hormones balanced.

When the simple starches in grains are balanced with the natural constituents of the whole grain that are sprouted, the negative hormonal effects of grains are diminished. However, with the exception of old-fashioned oatmeal and cracked rye berries, some individuals will need to keep their whole-grain intake down to only 25 percent of each meal. This will prevent reactions that diminish digestion and unbalance your hormones.

Legumes, Nuts, and Seeds

The legumes used in the recipes that follow should be soaked overnight to shorten cooking time and allow lower cooking temperatures. This also preserves melatonin and other hormones and vital phytochemicals that are easily destroyed by overcooking, and helps to minimize digestive problems.

Lentils, garbanzo beans (chickpeas), great Northern beans (Cannellini), and non-GMO soybeans are high in biologically active protein. When consumed as more than 50 percent of a meal, they will help to keep hormones balanced.

Nuts and seeds are powerfully concentrated sources of EFAs and protein. These nutrient-dense foods should be consumed in moderation, and in combination with other foods as in the recipes that follow. Avoid buying oil-roasted nuts or salted nuts, as their EFAs are low and protein is destroyed by roasting.

As with flours, legumes should be stored in tightly lidded jars in a dry, cool place, as moisture can make them stale and/or moldy.

Fish

The fish with the greatest concentration of EFA precursors to eicosanoid hormones are Arctic, Norwegian, or New Zealand Salmon; Arctic Mackerel; and Icelandic Cod or Haddock. The fatty acids in these fish are proven to lower blood cholesterol and triglyceride levels. Eating these fish can greatly benefit your heart and keep your circulatory system clean and healthy.

Despite the value of fish, a host of contamination issues make fish a food that must be purchased from reputable vendors who uphold high standards of purity. Fish from polluted waters should be avoided, as they can be contaminated with bacteria, parasites, mercury and heavy metals, and very toxic hormone blockers.

Most Atlantic salmon and local coastal fish are full of xenoestrogens and potential carcinogens, so limit your intake of fish unless they come from cleaner waters. New Zealand and Icelandic cold waters yield the best fish. The Arctic is probably the best source for salmon.

Fresh fish should not smell "fishy." The eyes of the fish should be clear, not cloudy, and the skin should be moist and shiny. Look for bruises, odd-colored edges, or spots—signs of old, decaying fish. Your fish dealer should be able to keep you informed about where and when fish were caught. Be aware that many markets sell fish that has been dipped in a solution of chlorine to retard spoilage. Chlorine is toxic and a potent hormone blocker.

Poultry and Beef

Poultry and beef are poor sources of energy-enhancing nutrients. The meat industry, with very few exceptions, uses hormones and antibiotics in raising live-stock, and poultry and beef are possible sources of bacterial contamination. The high saturated fat content of many meat products is also a cause of hormonal imbalances.

For those who want to keep animal protein in their diets, lean cuts of meats are an option. Best, however, is to consume meat sparingly, as a condiment to flavor a meal that is predominantly vegetables.

RECOMMENDED QUANTUM ENERGY FOODS

The following is a list and description of specially created Quantum Foods that you'll find included in many of the following recipes, or that you can add to your daily diet when you want to feel alert and energized or you are under extra-ordinary stress. These products are available from Quantum Energy Resources on the Internet (see the listing in the Resources section).

Multi-Nutra Food™

Multi-Nutra Food contains Japanese spirulina, stabilized rice bran and protein, bioactive peptides, wheatgrass, alfalfa, and royal jelly.

Coconut Butter

Use coconut butter in place of butter or margarine on sprouted toast or on your favorite hot cereal.

QuantaPollen™

Take this in between meals for quick energy and for keeping your immune system in tip-top shape.

Digeszyme™

This substance contains non-fungal enzymes to help with digestion. Use with each meal, especially if you are eating cooked food that is void of enzymes.

Quantum Salt™

This premium salt is from prehistoric salt beds. It is free of arsenic and pollutants and extremely rich in trace minerals.

Quantum Olive Oil™

This is the only solvent-free olive oil on the market that is truly cold-pressed and raw.

Quantum Sugar Crystals™

This raw cane sugar from Argentina does not contain any 2,4,5-T, a harmful dioxin derivative that diminishes your QEF.

Next, you will have an opportunity to put into practice all that you have learned. The following pages contain wonderful examples of the Quantum Energy Diet in action. Each recipe conforms to the Quantum Food guidelines, and each has been tested for the highest quality ingredients and taste potential. Enjoy!

QUANTUM FOOD RECIPES

Now that you have Quantum Foods in stock, and you know how to prepare them to achieve the best, most healthful effect, try some of the recipes on the following pages.

BREAKFAST RECIPES

SCRAMBLED TOFU

(SERVES 6)

3 eight-ounce non-GMO tofu cakes

2 tablespoons light miso

2 tablespoons *Quantum Coconut Butter*

1 cup mushrooms, sliced

$\frac{1}{4}$ cup olives, minced

1 medium tomato, seeded and chopped

1 tablespoon turmeric

$\frac{1}{4}$ teaspoon cayenne, or to taste

soy sauce to taste

$\frac{1}{2}$ cup fresh parsley, minced

2 green onions, sliced thinly

1. Place tofu cakes in a bowl with miso and mash together thoroughly. Set aside.

2. Heat butter in skillet and sauté mushrooms for a few minutes. Add tofu mixture, olives, tomatoes, and turmeric. Stir together well. Cover and simmer over low flame for five minutes.

3. Season to taste with cayenne and soy sauce. Sprinkle with parsley and green onions, and serve.

Variation: Add or substitute onion and garlic, carrot (diced or grated), and celery slices for variety. To vary flavor, add black pepper, nutritional yeast, thyme, and dill.

QuantaFood Supreme

(SERVES 1)

8 capsules *MultiNutraFood,* opened

4 tablespoons *QuantaFood*

3 capsules *QuantaPollen,* opened

1 cup *Bionaturae* Apricot, Pear, or Peach Nectar

1. Blend all of the ingredients in a blender until very smooth, about two minutes.

Cashew Cream Delight

(SERVES 2)

1 ½ cups raw cashews

1 cup water

1 cup fresh orange juice

½ cup raw sunflower seeds

1 teaspoon *Quantum Sugar Crystals*

1 cup fresh strawberries

1. Soak cashews in water and orange juice overnight in the refrigerator.

2. The next morning, blend all of the ingredients, except strawberries, in a blender until very smooth, about two minutes. Serve over fresh strawberries.

Almond Dream

(SERVES 2)

2 cups raw almonds

1 cup water

1 teaspoon vanilla

1 teaspoon *Quantum Sugar Crystals*

2 apples, diced into cubes

½ cup grated blanched almonds

1. Soak almonds overnight in water.

2. The next morning, blend almonds, water, vanilla, and sugar in a blender until very smooth, about two minutes. Serve over freshly diced apples. Top with almonds.

TOFU SUPREME

(SERVES 6)

¼ cup water

¼ cup tamari

½ teaspoon ground coriander seed

1 clove garlic, minced

2 packages or 3 blocks tofu (about 1 pound), cut into 1-inch squares

¼ cup arrowroot flour

1 tablespoon *Quantum Coconut Butter*

1 green onion, finely chopped

1. Mix water, tamari, coriander, and garlic together. Dip tofu cubes in mix and coat with arrowroot flour.

2. Heat butter in a wok or skillet, and fry tofu until golden. Drain well on paper towel. Garnish with finely chopped green onions.

HEARTY BREAKFAST RYE

(SERVES 6)

½ cup raisins

1 tablespoon grated lemon rind

½ teaspoon cinnamon powder

½ cup apple cider

3 cups cooked rye berries

½ cup raw pumpkin seeds

½ cup almonds, coarsely chopped and lightly roasted

1 tablespoon *Quantum Coconut Butter*

1. Simmer raisins, lemon rind, and cinnamon powder in apple cider for a few minutes, until raisins are plump.

2. Add cooked rye berries and simmer a few more minutes. Turn off heat.

3. Add pumpkin seeds, almonds, and coconut butter. Let stand covered for fifteen minutes or longer before serving.

APPLEBERRY SMOOTHIE

(SERVES 1)

1 cup fresh apple cider

½ cup strawberries or blueberries

1 fresh apple, diced

1 fresh pear, diced

4 capsules (opened) *Multi-Nutra Food*

½ cup soaked raw almonds

1. Place all of the ingredients in a blender, adding almonds last.

2. Blend for thirty seconds, or until creamy.

PINEAPPLE-CASHEW SMOOTHIE

(SERVES 1)

2 cups ripe pineapple chunks

1 cup water

½ cup presoaked cashews

½ frozen medium banana

4 capsules (opened) *Multi-Nutra Food*

1. Place all of the ingredients in a blender, adding cashews last.

2. Blend for thirty seconds, or until creamy.

ALMOND MILK SUPREME

(SERVES 1)

1 cup blanched raw almonds

2 cups water

1 teaspoon vanilla

1 teaspoon *Quantum Sugar Crystals*

1. Place almonds in a blender. Add 1 cup of the water and blend until smooth.

2. With blender running on high, add remaining water, vanilla, and sugar. Blend two minutes.

3. For smooth milk, strain the almond milk through cheesecloth over a bowl.

STEEL-CUT OATS

(SERVES 1)

4 cups water

1 cup oats

½ cup presoaked sunflower seeds

½ teaspoon cinnamon

1 teaspoon *Quantum Sugar Crystals*

2 tablespoon *Quantum Coconut Butter*

1. Bring the water to a boil. Slowly stir the oats into the boiling water. Return to a boil.

2. Reduce the heat to low, cover, and simmer until the water is absorbed, about forty-five minutes.

3. Mix sunflower seeds, cinnamon, and sugar into oatmeal. Top with coconut butter.

RYE-OAT PANCAKES

(SERVES 4)

1 cup whole rye flour

1 cup raw wheat germ

½ cup oat bran

2 cups water

2 tablespoons *Quantum Coconut Butter*

2 eggs or egg replacement

2 cups soy milk

1. In a mixing bowl, combine the flour, wheat germ, and oat bran.

2. Add water, butter, eggs, and soy milk. Stir vigorously until thoroughly combined.

3. Spoon on to hot griddle. When bubbles appear on the surface, flip over and cook for about three minutes.

LUNCH RECIPES

BURRITOS WITH PEPITAS

(SERVES 4)

3 tablespoons *Quantum Olive Oil*
1 clove of garlic, minced
½ cup chopped onions
1 jalapeno pepper
1 green bell pepper
1 cup green pumpkin seeds (pepitas), chopped
½ teaspoon cumin or turmeric
½ teaspoon coriander
1 teaspoon oregano
¼ teaspoon cayenne pepper
4 fresh basil leaves, chopped
1 mild green chili pepper
1½ cups cooked pinto beans
1 teaspoon *Quantum Salt*
1 tablespoon *Quantum Coconut Butter*
5 large flour tortillas
½ cup grated Monterey Jack cheese
¼ cup tomato juice

1. In a large skillet, heat oil over medium-high heat. Add garlic, onions, jalapeno peppers, green peppers, pumpkin seeds, cumin, coriander, oregano, and cayenne pepper. Sauté until vegetables are soft and the mixture is fragrant, about five minutes.

2. In a large bowl, mix together sautéed mixture and the remaining ingredients, except tortillas, cheese, and tomato juice.

3. Lay tortillas on a counter and divide bean mixture equally among them by placing it in log shapes on the edge of each tortilla. Sprinkle cheese on each bean log, then roll tortillas and use the back of a spoon to press in the filling on the sides.

4. Place burritos in same skillet used to cook the filling and pour tomato juice over them. Simmer until burritos are soft and juice has evaporated, about two minutes. Place burritos on a serving platter and serve hot.

SHIITAKE AND FRESH TOMATO SANDWICH

(SERVES 2)

6 large fresh shiitake mushrooms

2 tablespoons *Quantum Olive Oil*

1 ripe tomato, sliced

$\frac{1}{2}$ teaspoon of dried oregano

2 tablespoons fresh basil, minced

1 dash *Quantum Salt*, or to taste

1 dash cayenne pepper, or to taste

Four slices of sprouted whole-grain bread

1. Cut off stems of mushrooms and place in pan with olive oil. Cook at a low temperature until mushrooms are soft. Set aside.

2. Sprinkle tomato slices with oregano, basil, salt, and cayenne pepper.

3. Layer tomatoes and mushrooms between whole-grain bread slices.

Variation: Substitute four slices of zucchini or butternut squash for the mushrooms.

FENNEL-CABBAGE SUPREME

(SERVES 4)

3 tablespoons *Quantum Olive Oil*

$\frac{1}{2}$ teaspoon *Quantum Salt*

1 clove of garlic, minced

$\frac{1}{2}$ cup parsley, minced

2 tablespoons fennel seeds

1 scallion, minced

4 cups shredded cabbage

4 tablespoons crumbled goat cheese

1. In a large skillet, heat oil on medium-high heat. Add salt, garlic, parsley, fennel, scallions, and cabbage. Sauté for about five minutes.

2. Place cabbage mixture in a large serving bowl, sprinkle with goat cheese and serve hot.

QUANTUM CARROT SALAD

(SERVES 7)

6 cups shredded organic carrots

1 cup shredded organic green cabbage

½ cup finely chopped parsley

7 tablespoons *Quantum Olive Oil*

3 tablespoons *Quantum Coconut Butter*

Juice of 1 fresh lemon or 4 tablespoons *Bionaturae* Italian
Balsamic Vinegar

¼ teaspoon dried basil

½ teaspoon dried oregano

½ teaspoon cayenne pepper

1 teaspoon *Quantum Salt*

1. In a large bowl, combine carrots, cabbage, and parsley. Set aside.

2. In a small bowl, whisk together oil, butter, lemon juice or vinegar, basil, oregano, cayenne pepper, and salt.

3. Toss the dressing with the carrots and cabbage mixture. Serve at room temperature. Keeps for one week in the refrigerator.

PINE NUT SALAD

(SERVES 4)

2 heads romaine lettuce, washed and shredded

2 stalks celery, chopped

1 teaspoon *Quantum Salt*

4 tablespoons *Quantum Olive Oil*

½ cup pine nuts (pignoli nuts)

1. In a bowl, toss together lettuce and celery. Sprinkle with salt. Toss again, and allow to stand for twenty-five to thirty minutes.

2. Add the pine nuts and serve.

QUANTUM SALAD

(SERVES 4)

6 tablespoons *Quantum Olive Oil*

6 tablespoons fresh lemon juice

$\frac{1}{2}$ teaspoon basil

$\frac{1}{2}$ teaspoon oregano

$\frac{1}{2}$ teaspoon turmeric

1 teaspoon mustard

2 heads leaf lettuce, torn into bite-sized pieces

1 cup chopped spinach leaves

1 cup shredded carrots

1 cup diced broccoli

1 cup diced zucchini

1 cup diced celery

1 cup diced red pepper

1. In a small bowl, whisk together oil, lemon juice, basil, oregano, turmeric, and mustard. Set aside.

2. In a large bowl, toss the remaining ingredients together. Add dressing and toss again. Chill and serve.

Variation: Add a handful of one of the following to finished salad: raw sunflower seeds, tofu chunks, roasted soybeans, or grilled chicken.

VEGA RICE SALAD

(SERVES 4)

2 cups cooked basmati rice

1 cup fresh peas or sugar snap pea pods

1 scallion, minced

½ cup shredded fresh spinach

½ cup chopped parsley

2 tablespoons *Quantum Olive Oil*

2 tablespoons *Quantum Coconut Butter*

Juice of 1 fresh lemon

½ teaspoon dried oregano

½ teaspoon turmeric

1 teaspoon *Quantum Salt*

2 tablespoons mustard

1. In a large bowl, combine rice, peas or pea pods, scallions, spinach, and parsley. Set aside.

2. In a small bowl, whisk together olive oil, butter, fresh lemon juice, oregano, turmeric, salt, and mustard.

3. Toss the dressing with the rice mixture. Serve at room temperature.

MAIN MEAL RECIPES

MUSHROOM TOFU

(SERVES 3)

4 tablespoons *Quantum Olive Oil*
½ onion, diced
1 pound of non-GMO organic tofu
1 cup broccoli heads (frozen or fresh)
1 cup chopped fresh mushrooms
1 teaspoon *Quantum Salt*

1. Heat oil in small skillet.

2. Add all of the ingredients and sauté until vegetables are tender.

Variation: Serve over cooked millet, white basmati rice, or Bionaturae pasta.

TOMATO-ARTICHOKE SAUCE

(SERVES 8–10)

2 cups artichoke hearts
8 tablespoons *Quantum Olive Oil*
1 cup water
6 cups tomato puree
3 cups crushed tomatoes
2 garlic cloves
½ teaspoon basil
½ teaspoon oregano
1 teaspoon parsley
½ teaspoon marjoram
1 chopped onion
1 tablespoon VegaFood
1 teaspoon *Quantum Salt*

1. Cut artichoke hearts in four pieces. Place olive oil in a large saucepan. Simmer artichoke hearts at medium-heat for ten minutes.

2. Add all of the remaining ingredients. Cook for one to two hours over low heat. Serve over pasta.

BAKED DILL SALMON

(SERVES 3)

2 tablespoons mustard
1 teaspoon *Quantum Salt*
1 tablespoon lemon juice
3 salmon fillets
3 lemon slices
3 tomato slices
3 sprigs of fresh dill

1. Preheat the oven to 375°F.

2. In a medium-sized bowl, mix together mustard, salt, and lemon juice. Dip salmon fillets in mixture, coating both sides.

3. Place the fillets in large baking dish; place a lemon slice, a tomato slice, and a sprig of dill on top and cover.

4. Bake for about twenty minutes or until fish is cooked through.

Variation: Substitute cod or haddock for the salmon.

PESTO DELIGHT

(SERVES 2)

½ cup *Quantum Olive Oil*
2–3 cups fresh basil leaves
½ cup parsley, minced
¼ cup Romano Pecorino Cheese
1 teaspoon *Quantum Salt*
1 clove of garlic
½ cup pine nuts

1. Place olive oil in blender. Slowly add basil leaves and parsley to oil while blender is running.

2. Add remaining ingredients, except pine nuts, and blend mixture for about one minute. While blender is running, slowly add pine nuts and blend into a thick, creamy paste.

3. Serve over pasta or on whole-wheat pizza and top with additional Romano Pecorino grated cheese, as desired.

Tofu Meatless Loaf

(SERVES 6)

2 pounds organic non-GMO tofu

½ cup raw wheat germ

½ cup whole-grain rye flour

1 cup rolled oats

½ cup raw sunflower seeds

1 cup finely chopped parsley

2 tablespoons ketchup

2 tablespoons Dijon mustard

½ teaspoon garlic power

½ teaspoon thyme

½ onion, finely chopped

1 medium green pepper, finely chopped

4 tablespoons *Quantum Olive Oil*

1 teaspoon *Quantum Salt*

1. Preheat the oven to 350°F.

2. In a large bowl, crumble and mash tofu. Add all of the remaining ingredients and mix well.

3. Press mixture into an oiled loaf pan. Bake for one hour. Let cool ten minutes before removing from pan to slice.

Tofu Chop Suey

(SERVES 6)

4 tablespoons *Quantum Olive Oil*

1 teaspoon *Quantum Salt*

1 medium onion, chopped

1 slice of fresh ginger

1 clove garlic, minced

½ cup cabbage, sliced

1 medium carrot, sliced thinly

2 cups broccoli flowerets

1 green sweet pepper, diced

1 stalk celery, thinly sliced on the diagonal

1 pound tofu, in half inch cubes

2 tablespoon soy sauce

1 cup mung bean sprouts

1. In a large wok or pan, heat olive oil. Add salt, onion, ginger, garlic, and cabbage. Stir-fry for five minutes.

2. Add carrots, broccoli, green pepper, celery, and tofu. Cover pan and cook five minutes.

3. Add soy sauce and bean sprouts. Stir-fry until sauce is thickened. If desired, top with water chestnuts, and serve over rye berries or white basmati rice.

LENTIL CASSEROLE

(SERVES 6)

1 cup lentils

1 cup whole-wheat berries

2 cups water

1 cup chopped tomatoes

1 onion, chopped

½ cup chopped parsley

1 clove of garlic, minced

1 teaspoon *Quantum Salt*

1 teaspoon curry

4 tablespoons *Quantum Olive Oil*

1 teaspoon chili powder

1. Soak lentils and wheat berries in water overnight. Drain off water.

2. Preheat the oven to 300°F.

3. Bring two cups of water to a boil in a saucepan. Add lentils and wheat berries. Reduce heat and simmer for one hour until lentils and wheat berries are soft.

4. Stir in tomatoes, onion, parsley, garlic, salt, curry, oil, and chili powder, and place in a covered baking dish. Bake for thirty minutes.

BROCCOLI-NUT STIR-FRY

(SERVES 5)

2 large bunches broccoli (about 1 ½ pounds)

4 tablespoons *Quantum Olive Oil*

1 clove garlic, minced

3 tablespoons white wine

3 tablespoons natural soy sauce, or to taste

½ teaspoon freshly grated ginger

1 teaspoon *Quantum Salt*

½ cup coarsely chopped raw almonds

½ cup pine nuts

1. Wash and trim the broccoli. Slice the stems thinly and break the rest into slightly larger than bite-sized pieces. Set aside.

2. Heat the olive oil in a wok. Add the garlic, wine, soy sauce, ginger, and salt. Stir to mix.

3. Add the broccoli and stir until it is evenly coated with sauce. Stir-fry over moderately high heat until broccoli is bright green and tender crisp.

4. Stir in the almonds and pine nuts; stir-fry for another minute or so, then serve at once.

STUFFED PEPPERS ITALIANO

(SERVES 4)

2 large bell peppers

½ cup tomato sauce

2 cups cooked white basmati rice

4 tablespoons grated Romano Pecorino cheese

1 cup soft non-GMO tofu

½ cup raw wheat germ

2 teaspoons VegaFood

4 tablespoons of the chopped parsley

½ teaspoon oregano

1 teaspoon *Quantum Salt*

2 tablespoons *Quantum Coconut Butter*

1. Preheat the oven to 350°F.

2. Cut bell peppers in half lengthwise; remove seeds and membranes. Set aside.

3. In a large bowl, combine tomato sauce, rice, 2 tablespoons of the cheese, tofu, wheat germ, VegaFood, and 2 tablespoons of the chopped parsley. Blend together. If the mixture does not blend smoothly, add a little water.

4. Stuff the pepper halves with the mixture. Top with remaining grated cheese.

5. Bake until hot and cheese is melted, about ten minutes. Garnish with remaining parsley and serve.

MOUSSAKA

(SERVES 6)

2 large eggplants, in ¼-inch slices

4 tablespoons *Quantum Olive Oil*

2 tablespoons *Quantum Coconut Butter*

1 large onion, sliced into crescents

1 large tomato, peeled, seeded, and chopped

½ cup white wine (optional)

1 teaspoon *Quantum Salt*

1 cup cooked chickpeas

1 tablespoon oregano

3 tablespoons fresh basil

2 cups fresh spinach (chopped)

1 cup feta cheese, crumbled (optional)

1. Preheat the oven to 300°F. Bake eggplant for about fifteen minutes or until tender enough to be pierced with a fork. Do not turn off oven.

2. Heat olive oil and coconut butter in a skillet, and sauté onion until limp. Add tomato, wine, and salt. Cook uncovered for two to three minutes. Add chickpeas, oregano, and basil; cook a few minutes longer.

3. Place one layer of eggplant slices in bottom of a casserole dish, cover with a portion of the chickpea mixture and spinach. Sprinkle with some of the feta. Add another layer of eggplant and spinach. Top off with the remaining feta.

4. Cover and bake thirty minutes.

STUFFED ARTICHOKES

(SERVES 4–6)

4 whole large artichokes

2 cups fresh or dried bread crumbs

¼ cup Romano Pecorino cheese

1 teaspoon *Quantum Salt*

¼ cup fresh minced parsley

1 clove of garlic

½ cup white cooking wine

1-2 cups water

4 tablespoons *Quantum Olive Oil*

1. Wash artichokes; cut stems and trim the pointed edges ¼ of an inch down from the top of each artichoke. Soak artichokes and stems in cold water for one hour. Set aside.

2. In a large bowl, mix together bread crumbs, cheese, and salt. Add minced parsley. Squeeze garlic into bowl with a garlic presser and use a fork to press garlic into mixture evenly.

3. Place artichokes into a large pot. Stuff bread crumb mixture in and around artichoke leaves.

4. Drain and slice stems and add to the bottom of the pot along with wine. Add water until the artichokes are almost halfway covered with water. Put oil on the top of each artichoke.

5. Bring water to a boil. Cover pot and simmer on medium–low heat for one hour until center leaves are loose. Serve stuffed artichokes over Bionaturae pasta.

SESAME STRING BEANS

(SERVES 2)

2 pounds string beans, washed

½ cup water

¼ teaspoon soy sauce

4 tablespoons tahini

2 cups millet or pasta

1. Snap ends off string beans; break beans in half.

2. Place beans in a 3-quart saucepan with water; cover and simmer for five minutes. Add soy sauce and cook for ten minutes more.

3. Remove beans from heat and blend in the tahini. Spoon over individual servings of millet or pasta, and serve immediately.

STIR-FRY CHICKEN AND VEGGIES

(SERVES 4)

6 tablespoons *Quantum Olive Oil*

½ onion, minced

1 clove garlic, minced

1 large boneless chicken breast, cut into chunks

1 tablespoon finely minced fresh ginger root

2 cups diagonally sliced carrots

½ cup diagonally sliced celery

2 cups snow peas

2 cups broccoli florets

4 tablespoons water

¼ cup sliced water chestnuts

2 green onions, minced

½ cup raw wheat germ

1 cup bean sprouts

2 tablespoons soy sauce

1. Heat olive oil in a heavy wok. Sauté onion, garlic, chunks of chicken, and ginger root until chicken is browned.

2. Add carrots, celery, snow peas, and broccoli. Add 4 tablespoons water, cover, and cook for four minutes.

3. Add water chestnuts, green onions, wheat germ, and bean sprouts. Cook for another two minutes. Stir well while adding soy sauce.

Variation: Replace chicken with tofu or tempeh. Serve over white basmati rice or cooked wheat or rye berries.

ITALIAN-STYLE GREEN SOYBEANS

(SERVES 5)

1 large clove garlic, minced

2 cups sliced mushrooms

4 tablespoons *Quantum Olive Oil*

½ cup chopped parsley

1 teaspoon *Quantum Salt*

2 cups fresh green soybeans

1 teaspoon dried basil

½ teaspoon dried oregano

Pinch of tarragon

2 tablespoon wine vinegar

One 28-ounce can of imported plum tomatoes,
with liquid, crushed

¼ cup grated Romano cheese

2 pounds *Bionaturae* pasta

1. Sauté the garlic and mushrooms in the oil for two minutes. Add the parsley, salt, soybeans, basil, oregano, tarragon, vinegar, and tomatoes.

2. Cover and simmer for ten minutes; Stir in cheese. Simmer uncovered for ten minutes more.

3. Cook pasta during last ten minutes. Spoon the mixture over the pasta in a large bowl. Serve at once.

MILLET-PUMPKIN SEED CASSEROLE

(SERVES 4)

3 cups millet

4 tablespoons *Quantum Olive Oil*

1 medium onion, chopped

1 red bell pepper, chopped

7 stalks celery, chopped

½ cup raw pumpkin seeds, soaked and drained

5 cups water

1 teaspoon *Quantum Salt*

1. Wash and drain the millet. Place the millet in an iron skillet and dry roast, stirring constantly for five minutes; remove from heat. Set aside.

2. Heat the oil in a 3-quart saucepan over medium heat; add the onion and sauté for two to three minutes. Add pepper. Stir well. Add celery. Stir well.

3. Add millet to saucepan. Add pumpkin seeds, water, and salt. Bring to a boil. Reduce heat, cover, and simmer for forty minutes or until millet is soft.

SPINACH LASAGNA

(SERVES 6)

½ cup TVP (texturized vegetable protein)
1 cup water
1 pound *Bionaturae* lasagna noodles
2 pounds firm non-GMO tofu
1 cloves garlic, chopped
2 onions, chopped
1 cup fresh mushrooms
2 teaspoons oregano
1 teaspoon basil
½ teaspoon thyme
1 teaspoon *Quantum Salt*
1 32-ounce jar tomato sauce
1 pound spinach, steamed and chopped

1. Preheat the oven to 250°F.

2. Soak TVP for twenty minutes in water. Drain and set aside.

3. Cook lasagna noodles according to package directions.

4. In a large bowl, mix together tofu, garlic, onion, mushrooms, oregano, basil, thyme, and salt. Set aside.

5. Lay three lasagna noodles lengthwise on the bottom of a lightly oiled 9-by-13-inch pan. Spread on one-third of the tofu mixture. One-third of the tomato sauce, one-third of the spinach, and one-third of the TVP. Continue layering noodles with tofu mixture, sauce, spinach, and TVP.

6. Bake for thirty minutes.

SUNFLOWER EGGPLANT

(SERVES 5)

1 large eggplant (1 ½ to 2 pounds)

4 tablespoons *Quantum Olive Oil*

1 clove garlic, crushed or minced

⅓ cup water

1 teaspoon grated ginger

1 bunch scallions, chopped

2 tablespoons natural soy sauce or 1 teaspoon chili powder

1 teaspoon dry mustard

1 cup soaked raw sunflower seeds

1 teaspoon *Quantum Salt*

1. Peel the eggplant and slice into ¼-inch-thick slices. Cut the slices into pieces approximately ½-inch wide by 2-inches long.

2. Heat the oil in a large, heavy skillet. Add the eggplant, garlic, water, ginger, and scallions. Cover and simmer over low heat, stirring occasionally, until the eggplant is nearly tender. Add more water if necessary to keep the bottom of the skillet moist.

3. Add remaining ingredients and simmer until the eggplant is quite tender.

4. Stir in the sunflower seeds and serve at once as a side dish alone or over hot cooked grains.

ROASTED EGGPLANT ALMONDINE

(SERVES 3)

1 large eggplant (about 1 ½ pounds)

4 tablespoons *Quantum Olive Oil*

¼ cup raw almond butter

1 teaspoon *Quantum Salt*

1 clove garlic, crushed

Juice of ½ lemon

3 tablespoons finely minced parsley

½ teaspoon ground cumin

½ teaspoon ground coriander

Freshly ground pepper to taste

1. Preheat the oven to 400°F.

2. Brush the eggplant with olive oil.

3. Bake the eggplant whole, on a cookie sheet, for thirty to forty minutes, or until it has collapsed. Allow it to cool.

4. When the eggplant is cool enough to handle, peel off skin and drain off excess liquid. Mash with a fork and place in a serving container.

5. Add the remaining ingredients and stir together thoroughly. Serve with whole-grain cracker as an hors d'oeuvre.

SOUPS

YAM BEAN SOUP

(SERVES 6)

2 cups white cannellini beans

2 quarts of water

1 large yam cut into ½-inch squares

4 tablespoons miso paste

3 tablespoons *Quantum Olive Oil*

2 large carrots, grated

1 clove garlic, minced

1 cup minced onions

¼ teaspoon nutmeg or cinnamon

3 tablespoons minced parsley (garnish)

1. Soak beans overnight; drain off water.

2. Place beans in medium-sized pot with water, bring to a boil, and simmer for one hour.

3. Add remaining ingredients, except parsley; simmer for one hour more. Garnish with parsley.

ESCAROLE SOUP

(SERVES 2)

3 tablespoons *Quantum Olive Oil*

1 clove garlic, minced

2 bunches escarole, washed and sliced

1 teaspoon *Quantum Salt*

4 cups water

Soy sauce to taste

1. Heat the oil in a 2-quart soup pot. Add garlic, stirring briefly until garlic begins to brown.

2. Stir in escarole and salt. Cook over medium heat until the escarole wilts. Add the water and bring to a boil; then reduce heat, cover, and simmer for ten minutes.

3. Season to taste with soy sauce.

MILLET VEGETABLE SOUP

(SERVES 4)

2 cups Millet-Pumpkin Seed Casserole (see page 144)

2 cups baked zucchini, chopped

1 cup chopped onions

4 cups water

1 clove garlic, chopped

1 tablespoon soy sauce or to taste

4 teaspoons chopped parsley

1. Place the Millet-Pumpkin Seed Casserole, zucchini, onions, and water in a 2-quart soup pot. Bring to a boil, reduce heat, cover, and simmer for ten minutes.

2. Add garlic and soy sauce. Simmer for five minutes more. Ladle into bowls. Sprinkle a teaspoon of parsley on top of each serving.

GREEN BEAN SOUP

(SERVES 4)

3 tablespoons *Quantum Olive Oil*

1 cup minced celery

1 cup minced onion

1 cup minced carrots

1 clove garlic, minced

3 cups water

3 cups cut green beans

1 tablespoon soy sauce

$\frac{1}{2}$ teaspoon thyme

$\frac{1}{2}$ teaspoon oregano

$\frac{1}{2}$ teaspoon basil

3 medium tomatoes, peeled and chopped

1 cup cooked chickpeas, mashed

$\frac{1}{2}$ teaspoon *Quantum Salt*

2 tablespoons *Quantum Coconut Butter*

$\frac{1}{2}$ cup chopped parsley

1. Heat oil in a 4-quart saucepan over medium to low heat.

2. Add celery, onion, carrots, and garlic. Cook about five minutes until soft. Add water, green beans, and remaining ingredients, except parsley. Bring to a boil. Reduce heat; cover and simmer for fifteen minutes until green beans are tender.

3. Garnish with parsley.

CONDIMENTS, DIPS, AND SPREADS

CURRY DIP SUPREME

(YIELDS 2 CUPS)

1 cup plain yogurt or kefir

2 teaspoons curry powder

1 teaspoon turmeric

1 slice of raw ginger

¼ teaspoon chili powder

½ teaspoon *Quantum Salt*

1. Blend all of the ingredients in a blender until smooth.

2. Serve chilled with crudités or whole-grain crackers.

BLACK BEAN DIP

(SERVES 4)

6 ounces black turtle beans, cooked

1 large Bermuda onion

½ teaspoon chili powder

½ jalapeno pepper, sliced

½ teaspoon *Quantum Salt*

1 green pepper, chopped

1 large scallion, chopped

½ garlic clove, optional

1 teaspoon cumin

1 teaspoon paprika

2 teaspoons mustard

½ cup chopped parsley

4 tablespoons *Quantum Olive Oil*

1. Blend all of the ingredients in a blender until smooth, adding water if necessary to keep the mixture from becoming too thick.

2. Refrigerate in glass container until ready to use. Serve with tortilla chips or tacos.

DILLED MISO-TOFU DIP

(SERVES 4)

$\frac{1}{2}$ pound soft tofu

3 tablespoons mellow white miso

Juice of 1 small lemon

$\frac{1}{4}$ teaspoon garlic powder

3 tablespoons dill

$\frac{1}{4}$ teaspoon kelp powder, optional

$\frac{1}{4}$ cup soy milk

4 tablespoons *Quantum Olive Oil*

$\frac{1}{2}$ teaspoon *Quantum Salt*

1. Blend all of the ingredients in a blender until smooth.

2. Serve over organic sprouted bread.

CREAMY PARSLEY DRESSING

(SERVES 2)

2 ounces soft tofu

$\frac{1}{2}$ cup water

2 tablespoons lemon juice

2 tablespoons tahini

4 tablespoons *Quantum Olive Oil*

1 handful washed parsley

1 teaspoon baking powder

1 teaspoon *Quantum Salt*

1 teaspoon *Quantum Sugar Crystals*

$\frac{1}{2}$ teaspoon baking soda

$\frac{1}{2}$ teaspoon *Quantum Salt*

$\frac{1}{2}$ teaspoon vanilla

1. Place all of the ingredients in a blender and blend until creamy. Pour approximately $\frac{1}{4}$ cup of the dressing on four cups of your favorite salad. Toss well.

CHICKPEA SPREAD

(SERVES 3)

2 cups well-cooked chickpeas, mashed

1/4 cup minced green bell pepper

3 tablespoons minced fresh parsley

2 tablespoons minced scallions

Juice of 1/2 lemon

3 tablespoons sesame paste (tahini)

1/2 teaspoon dried dill

1/2 teaspoon cumin

1/4 teaspoon turmeric

1/2 teaspoon *Quantum Salt*

3 tablespoons *Quantum Olive Oil*

1. Place all of the ingredients in a bowl. Mix thoroughly.

2. Serve at once over celery sticks or with Swedish rye crisps.

SPINACH DIP

(YIELDS 2 CUPS)

12 ounces fresh spinach, washed and chopped

12 ounces of tofu

2 tablespoons fresh lemon juice

1 teaspoon oregano

1/2 teaspoon basil

1/2 teaspoon garlic powder

1 red bell pepper, chopped

4 tablespoons *Quantum Olive Oil*

1/2 teaspoon *Quantum Salt*

3 scallions or chives, finely chopped

1. Blend all of the ingredients, except scallions, in a blender until smooth.

2. Place dip in a small bowl and cover with finely chopped scallions or chives.

3. Serve with toasted sprouted bread.

Appendix

Common Toxic Commercial Product Ingredients and Potential Health Effects

Taking in food that is toxic to the system is one way, as we have seen, to abuse our bodies and lower our quantum energy fields. However, we can also bring toxins into the body through substances we breathe in and others we use in our daily lives, things like cleaners, deodorants, "beauty" products, and the like. This Appendix supplies you with a list of such potentially dangerous and toxic substances.

If you can find no substitute and must use the substances listed below, at least wear rubber gloves and/or a breathing mask. Also, be sure that the area is adequately ventilated.

I urge you to "detoxify" your home. Go through each room, beginning with the kitchen, and remove all toxicants, all substances on the following list. You may be surprised how enlightening reading a few labels can be, how dangerous your life has been, and how healthy it can be from now on.

COMMERCIAL ALL-PURPOSE CLEANERS

Avoid complex phosphates, chlorinated phosphates, morpholine, petroleum-based surfactants, dry bleach, kerosene, sodium bromide, glycol ether, Stoddard solvent, EDTA, and naphtha.

Chlorinated materials form organ-chlorine compounds and are stored in fat cells that can enter mothers' milk. Morpholine and glycol are potential liver and kidney toxins. Glycol ether, Stoddard solvent, naphtha, and kerosene are neuro-toxins that can cause confusion, headaches, lack of concentration, and other mental symptoms.

COMMERCIAL DEODORIZERS

Avoid methoxychlor, aromatic hydrocarbons, salicylates, petroleum distillates, formaldehyde, p-Dichlorobenzene, piperonal butxide, o-phenylphenl, and naphthalene.

Methoxychlor, dichlorobenzene, aromatic hydrocarbons, and naphthalene are potential neurotoxins, while salicylates may cause strong allergic or toxic reactions. Formaldehyde and piperonal butoxide are potential carcinogens.

COMMERCIAL DISH DETERGENTS

Avoid petroleum-based surfactants, naphtha, chloro-o-phenylphenol, germicides, diethanolamine, complex phosphates, and sodium nitrates.

Chlor-o-phenylphenol is toxic, while diethanolamine is a potential liver toxin. Naphtha is a neurotoxicant.

COMMERCIAL DISINFECTANTS

Do not purchase or use substances containing the following: naphtha, butyl cellosolve, chlorinated germicides, petroleum-based surfactants, sodium hypochlorite, sodium sulfite, or nitrite.

Naphtha is a neurotoxicant while butyl cellosolve and sodium nitrite is strong toxins.

COMMERCIAL FURNITURE POLISHES

Avoid petroleum-distillates, propellants, diglycol laurate, amyl acetate, petroleum-based waxes, and mineral spirits.

Diglycol laurate, amyl acetate, and mineral spirits are neurotoxins, while diglycol laurate is a potential liver and kidney poison. Mineral spirits contain the carcinogen benzene, and may cause lung and sinus irritation.

COMMERCIAL GLASS CLEANERS

Avoid organic solvents, petroleum-based waxes, complex phosphates, ammonia, phosphoric acid, alkyl phenoxy polyethoxy ethanols, naphtha, and butyl cellosolve.

Organic solvents, naphtha, and petroleum-based waxes are neurotoxins. When using organic solvents, beware of carcinogens such as benzene. Butyl cellosolve is a potential toxin. Phosphoric acid and ammonia are irritating and may disrupt DNA stability.

COMMERCIAL LAUNDRY DETERGENTS

Avoid petroleum-based surfactants of the aryl and alkyl group, tetra potassium pyrophospate, complex phosphates, fluosilicate, sodium toluene, xylene sulfonate, EDTA, optical brighteners, and benzethonium chloride.

Tetra potassium pyrophosphate is irritating and toxic while fluosilicate is a toxic pesticide. Benzethonium chloride is potentially toxic.

COMMERCIAL METAL POLISHERS

Avoid perchloroethylene, chromic acid, plasticizers, silver nitrate, phenolic derivative, kerosene, synthetic waxes, chromic acid, naphtha, and other organic solvents.

Perchloroethylene, kerosene, naphtha, chromic acid, and organic solvents are neurotoxins. Perchloroethylene is a potential carcinogen and is toxic to the kidneys and liver; exposure may be *fatal*. Silver nitrate is highly toxic and corrosive. Chromic acid is a liver and kidney toxin, and a possible carcinogen.

COMMERCIAL OVEN CLEANERS

Avoid ether-type solvents, petroleum distillates, methylene chloride, butyl cellosolve, and lye.

All of the above ingredients except lye are neurotoxins. Methylene chloride is a chlorinated hydrocarbon, which is stored in fatty tissue, and is a liver and kidney toxin. Lye is a corrosive poison. Ether-type solvents commonly contain the carcinogen benzene, which may lead to respiratory symptoms.

COMMERCIAL SPOT REMOVERS

Avoid p-hydroxybenzoic acid, oxalic acid, naphtha, benzene, perchloroethylene or trichloroethylene, sodium hypochlorite, hydrofluoric acid, aromatic petroleum solvents, aliphatic hydrocarbons, chlorinated hydrocarbons, or other petroleum hydrocarbons.

The ingredients listed above are extremely toxic to many parts of the body and contain suspected and known carcinogens, exposure to which can be fatal.

COMMERCIAL TOILET BOWL CLEANERS

Avoid complex phosphates, o- or p-Dichlorobenzene, chlorinated phenols, kerosene, salicylates, germicides, fungicides, 1, 3-Diochloro-5, sodium acid oxalate, and sodium acid sulfate.

Sodium acid oxalate, chlorinated phenols, and o- or p-Dichlorobenzene are highly toxic. Sodium acid sulfate is highly irritating and corrosive. Chlorinated phenols are corrosive, metabolic stimulants. Fungicides and germicides can be toxic and cause liver and kidney damage. O- or p-Dichlorobenzene is a liver and kidney poison and neurotoxicant.

REMEMBER

Do not purchase these toxicants in the first place. Go through your home and detoxify each room, one room at a time. Wrap each dangerous substance in newspaper and discard it carefully. Believe me, you and your family will be healthier and happier without them. However, if you must use these substances, take precautions such as wearing gloves, donning a breathing mask, and opening windows for adequate ventilation. Never take chances with your health.

Resources for Products and Further Information

This listing offers addresses and phone numbers and a brief note about product lines. Supplements should be taken under the direction of an alternative health-care practitioner, preferably one certified in Quantum Medicine. Some of these products require a physician's prescription, while others can be purchased in your local natural food store, by mail, or over the Internet. Addresses and phone numbers are subject to change.

QUANTUM FOODS, HEALTH PRODUCTS, AND RELATED PRODUCT LINES

A.C. Grace Company
1100 Quit Man Road
Big Sandy, TX 75755
903-636-4368
Their Unique E product is a superior form of vitamin E.

AltaDena
Industry, CA 91744
1-800-milk-123 (1-800-645-5123)
Manufacturer of raw (non-pasteurized) cheddar goat cheese and kefir. No colors or preservatives added. Certified rBST-free. Available in health food stores.

Bionaturae
Euro-USA Trading Co., Inc
North Franklin, CT 06254
www.bionaturae.com
Distributors of the only nontoxic fruit juices and jellies prepared with low heat to preserve nutrients and enzymes without American sugar or preservatives. Their Italian pasta is far superior to American grown grains, which may contain traces of mercury and are usually high in cancer-causing inorganic iron. Available in health food stores.

Chee Energy

P.O. Box 5009
Coeur d'Alene, ID 83814
888-263-9214 • Fax: 208-676-1880

Distributors of the hand-held LED device; Red Carpet Blanket, Energy Balancer (red, white, and blue) for balancing energy. They also sell a useful thermotherapy device.

Environmental Health Coalition of Western Massachusetts (EHCWM)

P.O. Box 614
Leverett, MA 01054

A grassroots organization created to help educate the public about environmental health issues and meet the needs of chemically injured people.

Lumiram Electric Corp.

White Plains, NY 10606
www.lumiram.com

Manufacturer and distributor of Chromalux full spectrum light bulbs.

Micro Essential Labs

P.O. Box 100824
Brooklyn, NY 11210
Customer Service: 718-692-3618

Manufacturers and suppliers of pH tape for home testing.

QuantumEnergy.com

200 Aaron Ct.
Kingston, NY 12401
Fax 845-340-8606
www.quantumenergy.com

Quantum Energy Resources is the exclusive source for Quantum Food formulations and products, for novel products for boosting immunity against viral invasion and mycoplasma, and for de-stressing the body with adaptogenic herbs. QE also has information on inexpensive EMF field protectors that work for cell phones, computers, televisions, and small electronic devices, and is a resource site for links to other manufacturers that sell EMF protection devices and nontoxic products.

Quantum Innovations

845-258-1288 • Fax 845-258-1298
kidsx3@warwick.net

This company is dedicated to bringing cutting-edge technology that when used with the principles of Quantum Medicine can bring the latest in nutritional support and patient wellness.

Products include:

QUANTUM LASER 5000: A small hand-held device that uses low level laser technology to reestablish Quantum Coherence (the coherent flow of biophotons).

MEDITHERM med2000: A convenient, portable IR camera that provides high resolution digital infrared thermal images. Highly accurate medical images can be made and stored. This technique allows a practitioner to objectively correlate and follow outcomes of treatment protocols on various clinical conditions.

QMSM: A newly improved light-weight and portable EAV device based on German technology to accurately detect organ-meridian dysfunction.

Light Beam Generator: A valuable tool for helping to restore proper functioning of the body's immune system defense by resisting toxic materials that may be blocking the lymphatic system.

SEMINARS AND LISTS OF CERTIFIED QUANTUM MEDICINE PRACTITIONERS

American Academy of Quantum Medicine

160 Correja Avenue
Iselin, NJ 08830-1433
Fax 732-283-0959
www.aaqm.org

The American Academy of Quantum Medicine offers certification seminars in Quantum Medicine and Quantum Nutrition. You can also contact the American Academy of Quantum Medicine for a list of Quantum Medicine practitioners in your area. This is a wonderful resource, especially for those who have health problems, or who just want to place themselves in the proper nutritional hands.

MANUFACTURERS AND SUPPLIERS OF COMMERCIAL HOUSEHOLD PRODUCTS WITH LOW TOXICITY

Arm & Hammer

Arm & Hammer Baking Soda
Church & Dwight CO. Inc. Dept CG
P.O. Box 7648
Princeton, NJ 08543-7648
Products available in supermarkets.

Bon Ami Company

Faultless Starch/Bon Ami Co.,
  Dept CG
1025 West 8th St.
Kansas City, MO 64101
Products available in supermarkets.

Earthrite

Earthrite, Dept CG
Corp. Center # 1
55 Federal Rd.
Danbury, CT 06813
203-731-5000
Nontoxic laundry detergents. Products available in health food stores.

E Magazine

28 Knight Street
Norwalk, CT 06881
An extraordinary magazine that focuses on toxic environmental issues and offers safe, nontoxic product ads and information.

EcoMall

P.O. Box 20553
Cherokee Station, NY 10021
212-535-1876
Features hundreds of environmentally friendly companies and products.

Ecoshop, Inc

Ecoshop, Inc.
5884 E. 82nd St.
Indianapolis, IN 46250
317-84-WORLD
Nontoxic household cleaners for home and office. Products available in health food stores.

Infinity Herbal

Infinity Herbal Products Dept. CG
Division of Jedmon Products Ltd.
Toronto, Canada M3J 3J9

Maker of Heavenly Horsetail All-Purpose Cleaner. Products available in health food stores.

Seventh Generation

Seventh Generation, Dept CG
Colchester, VT 05446-1672
800-456-1198

Low toxicity products for household cleaning. Products available in health food stores.

Recommended Reading for Keeping Your Home Nontoxic

Check the Internet for sources where you may purchase these valuable books, or consult your local library to find a copy. It will be well worth your time and effort.

Dadd, Debra Lynn, and Jeremy P. Tarcher. *The Nontoxic Home: Protecting Yourself and Your Family from Everyday Toxins and Health Hazards.* Revised edition, Ceres Press, Woodstock, NY, 1992.

Dadd, Debra Lynn, and Jeremy P. Tarcher. *Nontoxic and Natural: A Guide for Consumers; How to Avoid Dangerous Everyday Products and Buy or Make Safe Ones.* Ceres Press, Woodstock, NY, 1990.

Garland, Ann Witte. *For Our Kid's Sake: How to Protect Your Child Against Pesticides in Food,* New York, Mothers and Others for Pesticide Limits and the National Resources Defense Council, 1989.

Gosselin Robert, M.D., Ph.D., Roger P. Smith, Ph.D., Harold C. Holdge, Ph.D., and Jeanne Braddock. *Clinical Toxicology of Commercial Products,* 5th edition. Baltimore, MD: Williams and Wikins, 1984.

Bond-Berthold, Anne. *Clean & Green.* Woodstock, NY: Ceres Press, 1994.

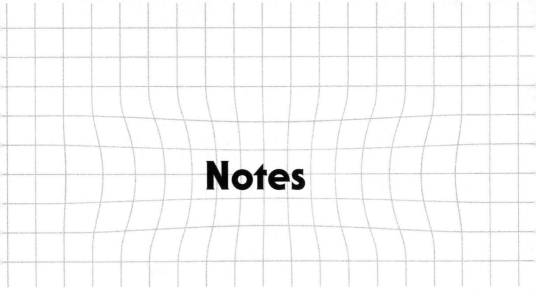

Notes

Even in a book, there is only so much information that will fit comfortably in a given chapter. There is so much more information available, and I know you must want to read in greater depth. These notes are designed to help you do that.

In this section, you will find research notes or references for each chapter. They are listed here to assist you who wish to investigate the concepts and ideas in greater depth. They are not listed in order of importance but generally follow the logic of each chapter.

I have provided as much information as possible, so you should be able to find these resources through the internet, at your local public library, and/or through the resources of college/university libraries in your area.

Chapter 1. The Birth of Quantum Medicine

Tegmark, M, Wheeler. "100 Years of Quantum Mysteries." *Scientific American* (September 2001): 68–75.

Yanick P. "Lymphatic Therapy for Chronic Immune & Metabolic Disorders, Detoxification and Successful Pain Elimination." *Townsend Letter for Doctors* (January 1995): 34–40.

Yanick P. "New Insights into Brain Fog, Memory & Learning Disorders, Insomnia, Anxiety, Depression and Immune Disorders." *Townsend Letter for Doctors & Patients* (June, 2000): 154–56.

Yanick P. "Hormone Resistance and the Ground Regulation System." *Townsend Letter for Doctors & Patients* (January 1999): 88–90.

Yanick, P. *Quantum Medicine.* Portland, OR: Writer Service Publications, 2000.

Yanick, P. *A Professional's Guidebook of Quantum Medicine.* Las Vegas, NV: American Academy of Quantum Medicine, 2001.

Popp, A. F. *New Avenues in Medicine in Bioresonance and Multiresonance Therapy.* H Brugemann, Ed. Brussels, Belgium: Haug, 1990.

Fiedler, N., et al. "A Controlled Comparison of Multiple Chemical Sensitivities and Chronic Fatigue Syndrome." *Psychosomatic Medicine* Vol. 58 (1996): 38–49.

Gruber, A. J, J. I. Hudson, and H. G. Pope, Jr. "The Management of Treatment-Resistant Depression in Disorders on the Interface of Psychiatry and Medicine: Fibromyalgia, Chronic Fatigue Syndrome,

Migraine, Irritable Bowel Syndrome, Atypical Facial Pain, and Premenstrual Dysphoric Disorder." *Psychiatric Clinicians of North America.* Vol. 19 (1996): 351–69.

Hudson, J. I., and H. G. Pope, Jr. "Fibromyalgia and Psychopathology: Is Fibromyalgia a Form of 'Affective Spectrum Disorder'?" *Journal of Rheumatology Supplement* Vol. 19 (1989): 15–22.

Hudson, J. I., et al. "Fibromyalgia and Major Affective Disorder: A Controlled Phenomenology and Family History Study." *American Journal of Psychiatry* Vol. 142 (1985): 441–6.

Walker E. A., et al. "Psychiatric Illness and Irritable Bowel Syndrome: A Comparison with Inflammatory Bowel Disease." *American Journal of Psychiatry* Vol. 147 (1990): 1656–61.

Simon, G. E, et al. "Immunologic, Psychological and Neuropsychological Factors in Multiple Chemical Sensitivity: A Controlled Study." *Annals of Internal Medicine* Vol. 119 (1997): 97–103.

Wood, G. C., R. P. Bentall, M. Gopfert, and R. H. Edwards. "A Comparative Psychiatric Assessment of Patients with Chronic Fatigue Syndrome and Muscle Disease." *Psychological Medicine* Vol. 21 (1991):619–28.

Balk, R. A. "Severe Sepsis and Septic Shock." *Critical Care Clinician* Vol. 16 (2000):179–192.

Sands K. E., et al. "Epidemiology of Sepsis Syndrome in Eight Academic Medical Centers." *JAMA* Vol. 278 (1997):234–240.

Yanick, P. "Food Supplement Benefits and Risks in Carcinogenesis: Part I." *Townsend Letter for Doctors & Patients* (Oct 2001).

Yanick, P. "Food Supplement Benefits and Risks in Carcinogenesis: Part II." *Townsend Letter for Doctors & Patients* (Dec 2001).

Yanick P. "Meridian/Organ Nutraceutic Resonant Complexes: New Hope for Chronically Sick Individuals." *Townsend Letter for Doctors & Patients* (May, 2000): 136–39.

Yanick, P. "Boosting Nutrient Uptake in Chronic Illness." *Townsend Letter for Doctors & Patients* (Dec 2000).

Yanick, P. "Biomolecular Nutrition and the GI Tract." *Townsend Letter for Doctors* (Dec., 1993).

Macleod, R. L. et al. "Inhibition of Intestinal Secretion by Rice." *Lancet.* Vol. 346 (1995): 90–92.

Gates, J. R., et al. "Association of Dietary Factors and Selected Plasma Variables with Sex-Hormone-Binding Globulin in Rural Chinese Women." *American Journal of Clinical Nutrition* Vol. 63.1 (1996): 22–31

Blobel, G., et al. "Metal Ion Chaperone Function of the Soluble Cu(I) Receptor Axis." *Science.* Vol. 278 (1997):853–56.

Yanick, P. "Dietary and Lifestyle Influences on Cochlear Disorders and Biochemical Status: A 12–month Study." *Journal of Applied Nutrition* Vol. 40, no. 2 (1988).

Gushleff, B. W. " The Role of Novel Phyto-Estrogen and Progestogen Therapy in the Menopausal Patient." *Informedica* Vol. 314 (1986): 205.

Yanick, P. "Physiological-Chemical Assessment of Undernutrition." *Townsend Letter for Doctors* (July, 1988): 285–88.

Yanick, P. "Biomolecular Nutrition and the GI Tract." *Townsend Letter for Doctors* (Dec. 1993):1248–1250.

Yanick, P. "Disorders of the Gall Bladder & Duodenum in Overweight Patients." *Townsend Letter for Doctors* (June 1994): 568–570.

Yanick, P. "Functional Correlates of pH in Accelerated Molecular and Tissue Aging." *Townsend Letter for Doctors* (May 1995): 34–39.

Yanick, P. "Functional Disturbances in Inner Ear Disorders." *Townsend Letter for Doctors* (August/September 1994): 860–863.

Yanick, P. "Chronic Fatigue Syndrome & Immunosuppression." *Townsend Letter for Doctors* (April 1994): 288–290.

Yanick, P. "Bioenergetic Regulation and Resiliency." *Explore* Vol. 4.5 (1993): 20–24.

Yanick, P. "Lymphatic Therapy for Chronic Immune & Metabolic Disorders, Detoxification and Successful Pain Management." *Townsend Letter for Doctors* (January 1995): 34–36.

Yanick, P. "MCS: Understanding Causitive Factors." *Townsend Letter for Doctors & Patients* (January 2001).

Yanick, P. "New Perspectives on Allergies & Seasonal Disorders." *Townsend Letter for Doctors & Patients* (May 2001).

Saltzman, J. R., et al. "Nutritional Consequences of Intestinal Bacterial Overgrowth." *Complete Therapy* Vol. 20.9 (1994):523–530.

Yanick P. "New Insights into Brain Fog, Memory & Learning Disorders, Insomnia, Anxiety, Depression and Immune Disorders." *Townsend Letter for Doctors & Patients* (June, 2000): 154–56.

Yanick P. "Hormone Resistance and the Ground Regulation System." *Townsend Letter for Doctors & Patients* (January 1999):88–90.

Gebbers, J. O., et al: Immunological Structures and Functions of the Gut." *Schweiz Arch Tierheilk.* Vol. 131 (1989): 221–238.

Kulli, P., et al. "Food Intolerance and Rheumatoid Arthritis." *Lancet* (1988): 1419–1420.

O'Farrelly, C., et al. "Association between Villous Atrophy in Arthritis and a Rheumatoid Factor and Gliadin-Specific IgG." *Lancet* (1988): 819–822.

Shanahan, F. A. "Gut Reaction: Lymphoepithelial Communication in the Intestine." *Science* Vol. 275 (1997):1897–1898.

Thedorou V., et al. "Integrative Neuroimmunology of the Digestive Tract." *Vet Res* Vol. 27 (1996): 427–442.

Wallace, J. L., et al. "Inflammatory Mediators in GI Defense and Injury." *PSEBM.* Vol. 214 (1997):192–203.

Fiocchi, C. "Cytokines and Intestinal Inflammation." *Transplant Processes* Vol. 18 (1996): 394–400.

Yanick, P. "Boosting Nutrient Uptake in Chronic Illness." *Townsend Letter for Doctors & Patients* (December 2000).

Adibi, S., and E. Phillips. "Evidence for Greater Absorption of Amino Acids from Peptide Than from Free Form in Human Intestine." *Clinical Research* Vol. 16 (1968): 446.

Craft, I. L., D. Geddes, C. W. Hyde, et al. "Absorption and Malabsorption of Glycine and Glycine Peptides in Man." *Gut* Vol 9 (1968) :425–437.

Adibi, S.A., M. R. Fogel, and R. M. Agrawal. "Comparison of Free Amino Acid and Dipeptide Absorption in the Jejunum of Sprue Patients." *Gastroenterology* Vol. 67 (1974): 586–591.

Reicht, G., W. Petritsch, A. Eherer, et al. "Jejunal Protein Absorption of Whey Protein and Its Hydrolysate." *JPEN* Vol. 16 (1992): 25S.

Neredith J. W., J. A. Ditesheim, and G. P. Zaloga. "Visceral Protein Levels in Trauma Patients Are Greater with Peptide Diet Than Intact Protein Diet." *J Trauma* Vol. 30 (1990):825–829.

Gardner, M.G. "Intestinal Assimilation of Intact Peptides and Proteins from the Diet, A Neglected Field." *Biol Rev* Vol. 59 (1984):289–331.

Boullin, D.J., R. F. Crampton, C. E. Heading , et al. "Intestinal Absorption of Dipeptides Containing Glycine, Phenylalanine, Proline, B-alanine, or Histidine in the Rat." *Clinical Science Molecular Medicine* Vol. 45 (1973):849–858.

Gardner, M.G. "Absorption of Intact Peptides: Studies on Transport of Protein Digest and Dipeptides across Rat Small Intestine in Vitro." *Q J Exp Physiol* Vol. 67 (1982):629–637.

Kontessis, P., S. Jones, R. Dodds, et al. "Renal, Metabolic and Hormonal Responses to Ingestion of Animal and Vegetable Proteins." *Kidney Int* Vol. 38 (1990):136–144.

Silk, D.B.A., P. D. Fairclough, M. L. Clark, et al. "Use of a Peptide Rather Than Free Amino Nitrogen Source in Chemically Defined 'Elemental' Diets." *JPEN* Vol. 4 (1980):548–553.

Keohane P.P., G. K. Grimble, B. Brown, et al. "Influence of Protein Composition and Hydrolysis Method on Intestinal Absorption of Protein in Man." *Gut* Vol. 26 (1985):907–913.

Webb, K.E. "Amino Acid and Peptide Absorption from the Gastrointestinal Tract." *Federation Proceeding* Vol. 45(1986): 2268–2271.

Amoss, M., J. Rivier, and R. Guillemin. "Release of Gonadotropins by Oral Administration of Synthetic LRF or a Tripeptide Fragment of LRF." *J Clin Endocrinol Metab* 35:175–177, 1972.

Bowers, C.Y., et al. "Porcine Thyrotrophin Releasing Hormone Is (Pyro)Glu-His-Pro(NH2)." *Endocrinology* Vol. 86 (1970): 1143–1153.

Gardner, M. L. G. "Entry of Peptides of Dietary Origin into the Circulation." *Nutrition and Health* Vol. 2 (1983):163–171.

Adibi, S.A. "Intestinal Absorption of Dipeptides in Man: Relative Importance of Hydrolysis and Intact Absorption." *Journal of Clinical Investigation* Vol. 50 (1971): 2266–2275.

Newey, H., and D. H. Smyth. "The Intestinal Absorption of Some Dipeptides." *Journal of Physiology* Vol. 145 (1959): 48–56.

Yanick, P *Quantum Medicine*. Portland, Oregon: Writer Service Publications, 2000.

Yanick, P *A Professional's Guidebook of Quantum Medicine,* American Academy of Quantum Medicine, Las Vegas, NV, 2001.

Popp, A. F. "New Avenues in Medicine," in *Bioresonance and Multiresonance Therapy.* H Brugemann, Ed. Brussels, Belgium: Haug, 2000.

Balk, R. A. *Critical Care Clinics.* Vol. 16 (2000): 179–92.

Chapter 2. The Scientific Validation of Quantum Medicine

Burr H. S. *Transactions of the American Neurology Association* Vol. 63 (1939).

Burr H. S. *American Journal of Obstretics and Gynecology* (1942): 44.

Burr H. S. *Blueprint for Immortality: The Electric Patterns of Life.* Saffron Walden: CW Daniel,1972.

Burr H. S. *Yale Journal of Biological Medicine* (1944): 16.

Burr H. S. *Proceedings of National Academy of Science* (1946): 32.

Burr H. S. *Yale Journal of Biological Medicine* (1945): 17.

Burr H. S. *Federal Proceedings* (1947): 6.

Burr H. S. *Yale Journal of Biological Medicine* (1942): 14.

Burr H. S. *Yale Journal of Biological Medicine,* (1947):19.

Burr H. S. *Yale Journal of Biological Medicine* (1949): 21.

Abrams A *New Concepts in Diagnosis and Treatment.* San Francisco: Philopolis Press, 1916.

Boyd, W. *Royal Society of Medicine,* 1925.

Becker, R. O. *Cross Currents: The Perils of Electropollution.* Putnam. NY: Tarcher, 1990.

Lakhovsky, G. *The Secret of Life.* Sussex, England: True Health Publishing, 1951.

Crile, G. *The Phenomena of Life: A Radio-electric Interpretation.* 1936.

Lewis, T. *British Medical Journal* Vol. 431 (1937).

Hunt, V. *Progress Report: A Study of Structural Integration from Neuromuscular Energy Field and Emotional Approaches.* Los Angeles, CA: UCLA, 1977.

Kirlian, S. *Kirlian Photography.* Russia., 1949

Mandell, P. *Energy Emission Analysis.* EV Publishing, 1988.

DeVernejourl, P. *The Kirlian Aura.* New York: Doubleday, 1974.

DeVernejourl, P. "The Kirlian Question." *Bulletin of the Academy of National Medicine* (1985).

Kim, P. *Design for Destiny.* New York, NY: Ballantine Books, 1974.

Tiller, W. *Energy Field Observations.* 1988.

Motoyama, H. *Science and the Evolution of Consciousness.* Autumn Press, 1978.

Voll, R. *American Acupuncture* Vol. 8. (1980).

Yanick, P. *Quantum Medicine.* Portland, OR: Writer Service Publications, 2000.

Yanick, P. *A Professional's Guidebook of Quantum Medicine.* Las Vegas, NV: American Academy of Quantum Medicine, 2001.

Yanick, P. *Manual of Neurohormonal Regulation.* Coldbrook, VT: Biological Energetic Press, 1992.

Yanick, P. *Biological Energetic Regulation Method.* Coldbrook, VT: Biological Energetic Press, 1992.

Yanick, P. *Bioregulation, Regeneration and Lifespan Extension.* Yanick, Inc. 1994.

Smith, J. *The Dimensions of Healing: A Symposium* The Academy of Parapsychology and Medicine, 1972.

Hunt, V. *Science of Mind,* 1982.

Chapter 3. The Body's Incredible Innate Healing Powers

Reynonds, R. J. "The Gas Between the Stars." *Scientific American* (2001): 34–43.

Ferriere, K. M. in *Reviews in Modern Physics* Vol. 73 (2001): 4.

Stoicheff, H., and C. Vital. "Mitochondrial DNA and Disease." *New England Journal of Medicine* Vol. 334.4 (1996): 270–271.

Wallace, D. C. "Mitochondrial DNA in Aging and Disease." *Scientific American* (1997): 40–47.

Richter, C. "Oxidative Damage to Mitochondrial DNA and Its Relationship to Aging. *Int J Biochem Cell Biol* Vol. 27.7 (1995): 647–653.

Yanick, P. "Functional Correlates of pH in Accelerated Molecular and Tissue Aging." *Townsend Letter for Doctors,* May, 1995.

Blaylock, R. L. A "Review of Conventional Cancer Prevention and Treatment and the Adjunctive Use of Nutraceutical Supplements and Antioxidants. Is There Danger or Significant Benefit?" *JAMA* Vol. 3.3 (2000): 17–35.

Loft, S., et al. "Cancer Risk and Oxidative DNA Damage in Man." *J Mol Med.* Vol. 74 (1996): 297–312.

Wei, Q., et al. "DNA Repair: A Potential Marker for Cancer Susceptibility." *Cancer Bulletin* Vol. 46 (1994): 233–37.

Legerski, R. J., et al. "DNA Repair Capability and Cancer Risk." *Cancer Bulletin* Vol. 46 (1994): 228–32.

Noroozi, M., et al. "Effects of Flavonoids and Vitamin C on Oxidative DNA Damage to Human Lymphocytes." *American Journal of Clinical Nutrition* Vol. 67 (1998): 1210–18.

Wei, Y. H., and S. H. Dao. "Mitochondrial DNA Mutations and Lipid Peroxidation in Human Aging." In C. D. Berdainer and J. L. Hargrove, *Nutrients and Gene Expression.* Boca Raton: CRC Press, 1996.

Rucker, R, and D. Tinker. "The Role of Nutrition in Gene Expression: A Fertile Field for the Application of Molecular Biology." *Journal of Nutrition* Vol. 116 (1986): 177–189.

Yanick, P. *Quantum Medicine.* Portland, OR: Writer Service Publications, 2000.

Yanick, P *A Professional's Guidebook of Quantum Medicine.* Las Vegas, NV: American Academy of Quantum Medicine, 2001.

Popp, A. F. "New Avenues in Medicine" in *Bioresonance and Multiresonance Therapy,* H. Brugemann (Ed.). Brussels, Belgium: Haug, 1990.

DeVernejourl, P. *The Kirilian Aura.* New York: Doubleday, 1974.

Zimmerman, J. *Psychosomatic Medicine* 1979:11.

Hunt, V. *Brain Mind Bulletin* Vol. 3 (1978): 9.

Popp, F. A., et al. "Biophotonic Emission of the Human Body." *J Photochem & Photobiol,* Vol. 40 (1997): 187–89.

Popp, F. A., and J. J. Chang. "Mechanism of Interaction between Electromagnetic Fields and Living Systems." *Science in China* Vol. 43 (2000): 507–18.

Rettemyer, M., A. F. Popp, and W. Nagl. *Naturwissenchaften* Vol. 11 (1981): 572–3.

Benveniste, J. Letter. *The Lancet* (1998): 351.

Benveniste, J., et al. "A Simple Fast Method for *In Vivo* Demonstration of Electromagnetic Molecular Signaling (EMD) via High Dilution or Computer Recording." *FASEB Journal* Vol. 13 (1999): A163.

Burr, H. S. *The Fields of Life.* New York: Ballantine, 1972.

Gerber, R. *Vibrational Medicine.* Santa Fe: Bear and Company, 1988.

Chapter 4. DNA and Oxidative Stress: Aging and Cancer

Jensen, B., and M. Anderson. *Empty Harvest.* Garden City Park, NY: Avery, 1990.

"Veggie Nutrients Dip in Tests." *Omaha World-Herald* January 29, 2000: 6.

Finely, J., et al. "Selenium Content of Foods Purchased in North Dakota." *Nutr. Res.* Vol. 16 (1996): 723–28.

World Cancer Research Fund. *Food, Nutrition and the Prevention of Cancer. A Global Perspective.* Washington, DC: American Institute for Cancer Research,1997.

See, D. *Journal of the American Nutraceutical Association* Vol 2(1999): 25–41.

Yanick, P. "Food Supplement Benefits and Risks in Carcinogenesis: Part I." *Townsend Letter for Doctors & Patients.* Oct., 2001.

Block, J. B., and S. Evans. "Clinical Evidence Supporting Cancer Risk Reduction with Antioxidants and Implications for Diets and Supplements. *JAMA.* Vol. 3.3 (2000): 6–16.

Yanick, P. "Food Supplement Benefits and Risks in Carcinogenesis: Part II." *Townsend Letter for Doctors & Patients,* Dec 2001.

Heber, D. *What Color is Your Diet?* New York: HarperCollins, 2001.

Houston, M.D., and J. S. Strupp. "Prevention and Treatment of Cancer: Is the Cure in the Produce Aisle?" *JAMA*. Vol. 3.3 (2000): 27–30.

Reed, M. J., and A. Purohit. "Breast Cancer and the Role of Cytokines in Regulating Estrogen Synthesis." *Endocrine Review* Vol. 18 (1997): 701–715.

Stoicheff, H., and C. Vital. "Mitochondrial DNA and Disease." *N Eng J Med* Vol. 334.4 (1996): 270–271.

Wallace, D.C. "Mitochondrial DNA in Aging and Disease." *Scientific American* (1997): 40–47.

Richter, C. "Oxidative Damage to Mitochondrial DNA and Its Relationship to Aging." *Int J Biochem Cell Biol* Vol 27.7 (1995): 647–653.

Yanick P. "Functional Correlates of pH in Accelerated Molecular and Tissue Aging." *Townsend Letter for Doctors,* May, 1995.

Blaylock, R. L. "A Review of Conventional Cancer Prevention and Treatment and the Adjunctive Use of Nutraceutical Supplements and Antioxidants. Is There Danger or Significant Benefit?" *JAMA*. Vol. 3.3 (2000): 17–35.

Loft, S., et al. "Cancer Risk and Oxidative DNA Damage in Man." *J Mol Med*. Vol. 74 (1996): 297–312.

Wei, Q., et al. "DNA repair: A Potential Marker for Cancer Susceptibility." *Cancer Bulletin* Vol. 46 (1994): 233–37.

Chapter 5. pH for Health and Energy

Mountcastle, V. *Textbook of Medical Physiology,* St. Louis: C.V. Mosby, 1980.

Yanick, P., and R. Jaffee. *Clinical Chemistry and Nutrition: A Physician's Desk Reference*. Coldbrook, VT: Biological Energetic Press, 1988.

Yanick, P. "Physiological-Chemical Assessment of Undernutrition." *Townsend Letter for Doctors,* July, 1988.

Yanick, P. "Functional Correlates of pH in Accelerated Molecular and Tissue Aging." *Townsend Letter for Doctors,* May, 1995.

Brahmi, Z., et al. "The Effect of Acute Exercise on NK Cell Activity of Trained and Sedentary Human Subjects." *J Clin Immunol* Vol. 5 (1985): 321–28.

Wolfgang, I., in *Umweltmedizin*. Ed. by J. Trevin and W. Taalkenhammer. Idstein, Germany: Mowe-Verlag, 1991.

Engler, I. *Water.* Termington, Germany: Sommer-Verlag, 1991.

Grander, J. and Schauberger, V. *On the Track of Water's Secrets*. Vienna, Austria: Uranus, 1995.

Will, R. *Geheimnis Wasser.* Munich, Germany: Knaur-Verlag, 1993.

Yanick, P. "Experiments with Water during Various Detoxification Protocols." Unpublished Manuscript, 2001.

Yanick P. Detoxification Breakthroughs for Allergies and Chronic Toxicity." *Townsend Letter for Doctors and Patients.* July 2001.

Yanick, P. *A Professional's Guidebook to Quantum Medicine.* Las Vegas, NV: American Academy of Quantum Medicine, 2001.

Yanick P. "Meridian/Organ Nutraceutic Resonant Complexes: New Hope for Chronically-Sick Individuals." *Townsend Letter for Doctors & Patients* (May, 2000): 136–39.

Yanick P. *Quantum Medicine.* Portland, OR: Writer Service Publications, 2000.

Yanick, P. "Boosting Nutrient Uptake in Chronic Illness." *Townsend Letter for Doctors & Patients,* December 2000.

Yanick, P. "Functional Medicine Update." *Townsend Letter for Doctors,* Feb., 1994.

Yanick, P. *Bioregulation, Regeneration and Lifespan Extension.* Yanick, Inc. 1994.

Coburn, T., et al. *Our Stolen Future.* New York, NY: Penguin, 1996.

Labrie, C, A. Belanger, and F. Labrie. "Androgenic Activity of Dehydroepiandrosterone and Androstenedione in the Rat Ventral Prostate". *Endocrinology* Vol. 123 (1988): 1412–1417.

Labrie F. "Intracrinology." *Mol Cell Endocrinol.* Vol. 78 (1991): C113–C118.

Roy, R., and A. Belanger. "Lipoproteins: Carriers of Dehydroepiandrosterone Fatty Acid Esters in Human Serum." *J Steroid Biochem* Vol. 34 (1989): 559–561.

Provencher, P. H., R. Roy, and A. Belanger. "Pregnenolone Fatty Acid Esters Incorporated into Lipoproteins: Substrates in Adrenal Steroidogenesis." *Endocrinology* Vol. 130 (1992): 2717–2724.

Roy, R., and A. Belanger. "Formation of Lipoidal Steroids in Follicular Fluid." *J Steroid Biochem* Vol. 33 (1989): 257–262.

Labrie, F., A. Dupont, and A. Belanger. "Complete Androgen Blockade for the Treatment of Prostate Cancer." In: V. T. De Vita, S. Hellman, and S. A. Rosenberg, Eds. *Important Advances in Oncology.* Philadelphia, Lippincott: 1985.

Brochu, M, et al. "Effects of Flutamide and Aminoglutethimide on Plasma 5a-reduced Steroid Glucuronide Concentrations in Castrated Patients with Cancer of the Prostate." *J Steroid Biochem* Vol. 28 (1987): 619–622.

Belanger, A., et al. "Steroid Glucuronides: Human Circulatory Levels and Formation by LNCaP Cells." *J Steroid Biochem Mol Biol* Vol.40 (1989): 593–598 .

Labrie, F., et al. "Structure, Function and Tissue-specific Gene Expression of 3b-hydroxysteroid Dehydrogenase/5–ene-4–ene Isomerase Enzymes in Classical and Peripheral Intracrine Steroidogenic Tissues." *J Steroid Biochem Mol Biol* Vol. 43 (1992): 805–826.

Yanick, P. "New Insights into Brain Fog, Memory & Learning Disorders, Insomnia, Anxiety, Depression and Immune Disorders." *Townsend Letter for Doctors & Patients* (June, 2000): 154–56.

Yanick, P. "Hormone Resistance and the Ground Regulation System." *Townsend Letter for Doctors & Patients* (January 1999): 88–90.

Yanick, P. *Quantum Medicine.* Portland, OR: Writer Service Publications, 2000.

Yanick, P. *A Professional's Guidebook of Quantum Medicine.* Las Vegas, NV: American Academy of Quantum Medicine, 2001.

Yanick, P., and V. Giampapa. *ProHormone Nutrition.* Montclair, NJ: Longevity Institute International, 1998

Yanick, P., and V. Giampapa. *Quantum Longevity.* Los Angeles, CA: Promotion Publishing, 1997.

Chapter 6. Environmental Toxins: The Dangers and How to Avoid Them

Wolfe, M. S., et al. "Blood Levels of Organochlorine Residues and Risk of Breast Cancer." *J Natl Cancer Inst* Vol. 85.8 (1993): 468–652.

Coburn, T., et al. *Our Stolen Future.* New York: Penguin, 1996.

Chapter 7. Nature's Healing Foods: Phytochemicals

Coburn, T., et al. *Our Stolen Future.* New York: Penguin, 1996.

Stoicheff, H., and C. Vital. "Mitochondrial DNA and Disease." *N Eng J Med* Vol. 196 (1996): 270–271.

Wallace, D. C. "Mitochondrial DNA in Aging and Disease." *Scientific American* (1997): 40–47.

Richter, C. "Oxidative Damage to Mitochondrial DNA and Its Relationship to Aging." *Int J Biochem Cell Biol* Vol. 27.7 (1995): 647–653.

Yanick, P. "Functional Correlates of pH in Accelerated Molecular and Tissue Aging." *Townsend Letter for Doctors,* May, 1995.

Blaylock, R. L. "A Review of Conventional Cancer Prevention and Treatment and the Adjunctive Use of Nutraceutical Supplements and Antioxidants. Is there Danger or Significant Benefit?" *JAMA.* Vol. 3.3 (2000): 17–35.

Loft, S., et al. "Cancer Risk and Oxidative DNA Damage in Man." *J Mol Med.* Vol. 74 (1996): 297–312.

Wei, Q., et al. "DNA Repair: A Potential Marker for Cancer Susceptibility." *Cancer Bulletin.* Vol. 46 (1994): 233–37.

Legerski, R. J., et al. "DNA Repair Capability and Cancer Risk." *Cancer Bulletin.* Vol. 46 (1994): 228–32.

Noroozi, M., et al "Effects of Flavonoids and Vitamin C on Oxidative DNA Damage to Human Lymphocytes." *Am J Clin Nutr.* Vol. 67 (1998): 1210–18.

Wei, Y. H., and S. H. Dao. "Mitochondrial DNA Mutations and Lipid Peroxidation in Human Aging." In C. D. Berdainer and J. L. Hargrove. *Nutrients and Gene Expression.* Boca Raton, FL: CRC Press, 1996.

Rucker, R., and D. Tinker. "The Role of Nutrition in Gene Expression: A Fertile Field for the Application of Molecular Biology." *J Nutr* Vol. 116 (1986): 177–189.

Yanick, P. *Manual of Neurohormonal Regulation.* Coldbrook, VT: Biological Energetic Press, 1992.

Becker, R. O. *Cross Currents: The Perils of Electropollution.* Putnam, NY: Tarcher, 1990.

Gillette, B. "Raising the Alarm: Concerns Linger About EMFs." *E Magazine,* Nov-Dec (2001): 40–41.

Jensen, B, and M. Anderson. *Empty Harvest.* Garden City Park, New York: Avery, 1990.

"Veggie Nutrients Dip in Tests." *Omaha World-Herald,* January 29 (2000): 6.

Finely, J. et al: "Selenium Content of Foods Purchased in North Dakota." *Nutr. Res.* Vol. 16 (1996): 723–728.

World Cancer Research Fund. *Food, Nutrition and the Prevention of Cancer. A Global Perspective.* Washington, D.C.: American Institute for Cancer Research, 1997.

Hu, J., et al. "Risk Factors for Oesophageal Cancer in Northeast China." *Int J Cancer* Vol. 57 (1994): 38–46.

Haung, M. T., et al. "Inhibition of Skin Tumorgenesis by Rosemary and its Constituents Carnosol and Ursolic Acid." *Cancer Res.* Vol. 54 (1994): 701–8.

Steinmetz, K. A., et al. "Vegetables, Fruit, and Cancer Prevention: A Review." *J Am Diet Assoc.* Vol. 96 (1996): 27–37.

Winter, J., et al. *Chemicals in the Human Food Chain.* New York: Van Nostrand Reinhold, 1990.

World Health Organization. *Report on the Panel on Food and Agriculture.* Geneva, Switzerland: World Health Organization, 1992.

Minchin, R. F., et al. "Role of Acetylation in Colorectal Cancer." *Mutat Res.* Vol. 290 (1993): 35–42.

Sinha, R., et al. "High Concentrations of the Carcinogen 2–amino-1–methel-6–phenykunudazi Occur in Chicken but Are Dependent on the Cooking Method." *Cancer Res.* Vol. 55 (1996): 16–19.

Snyderwibe, E. G. "Some Perspective on the Nutritional Aspects of Breast Cancer Research. Food Derived HCAs as Etiologic Agents in Human Mammary Cancer." *Cancer* Vol. 74 (1994): 977–94.

Sacarello, H. L. A. *Handbook of Hazardous Materials.* Washington, DC: 1994. Lewis Publishers, 1994.

Yanick, P. "Food Supplement Benefits and Risks in Carcinogenesis: Part I." *Townsend Letter for Doctors & Patients,* Oct., 2001.

Yanick, P. "Food Supplement Benefits and Risks in Carcinogenesis: Part II. *Townsend Letter for Doctors & Patients,* Dec., 2001.

Heber, D. *What Color is Your Diet?* New York: HarperCollins, 2001.

Houston, M. D., and J. S. Strupp. "Prevention and Treatment of Cancer: Is the Cure in the Produce Aisle?" *JAMA* Vol. 3.3 (2000): 27–30.

Block, J. B., and S. Evans. "Clinical Evidence Supporting Cancer Risk Reduction with Antioxidants and Implications for Diets and Supplements." *JAMA.* Vol. 3.3 (2000): 6–16.

Chapter 8. Combating Viral Infections and Mycotoxins

Auernhammer, C.J., et al. "Effect of Growth Hormone and Insulinlike Growth Factor I on the Immune System." *Eur. J. Endocrinology.* Vol. 133 (1995): 635–45.

Rudman, D; et. al. "Effect of Human Growth Hormone in Men over 60 Years Old." *N.* Eng. J. Med. *Vol. 323 (1990):1–9.*

Loh, E., and J. L. Swain. "Growth Hormone for Heart Failure-Cautious Optimism." N. Eng. J. Med. Vol. 334 (1996): E856–57.

Wolthers, T; G. Thorbjorn, and J. O. Lunde. "Effect of G. H. Administration on Functional Hepatic Nitrogen Clearance: Studies in Normal Subjects and G. H. Deficient Patients." *J. Clin. Endocr. Metab.* Vol. 78 (1994): 1220–24.

Rosen, T., et al. "Consequences of Growth Hormone Deficiency in Adults and the Benefits and Risks of Recombinant Human Growth Hormone." *Horm. Res.* Vol. 43 (1995): 93–99.

Rosen, T., et. al. "Cardiovascular Risk Factors in Adult Patients with Growth Hormone Deficiency." *Acta Endocrin* Vol. 129 (1993):195–200.

Papadeakis, M.A., et. al. "Growth Hormone Replacement in Healthy Older Men Improves Body Composition but not Functional Ability." *Annals of Internal Medicine* Vol. 124 (1996):708–16.

Mukherjee, T. M., K. Smith, and K. Maros. "Abnormal Red-cell Morphology in Myalgic Encephalomyelitis." *Lancet* Vol. 2 (1987): 328–329.

Arnold, D. I., et al. "Excessive Intracellular Acidosis of Skeletal Muscle on Exercise in a Patient with a Post-viral Exhaustion/Fatigue Syndrome." *Lancet* Vol. 1 (1984): 1367–68.

Buist, Robert A. *Journal of Orthomolecular Med.* Vol. 3.3 (1988).

Behan, P. O., W. M. H. Behan, and E. J. Bell. "The Post-viral Fatigue Syndrome-Analysis of Findings in Fifty Cases." *Journal of Infections* Vol. 10 (1985): 211–222.

Cox, I.M., et al. "RBC Magnesium and Chronic Fatigue Syndrome." *Lancet* Vol. 337 (1991): March 30.

Perger, F. "Klinik der Lambliasis Intestinalis und Ihre Verbreitung in Mittleleuropa." *Nautramed* Vol. 3, 1988.

Galland, L. "Leaky Gut Syndromes." *Townsend Letter for Doctors.* Aug/Sept, 1995.

Masoro, E. J. "Food Restriction in Rodents: An Evaluation of Its Role in the Study of Aging." *Journal of Gerontology.* Vol. 43 (1988): B59–B64.

Gates, J. *Cornell University Study.* Manuscript in Publication, 2002.

Wyatt, J., et al. "International Permeability and the Prediction of Release in Crohn's Disease." *Lancet* Vol. 341 (1993): 1437–9.

Gulbins, E., and F. Lang. "Pathogens, Host-Cell Invasion and Disease." *American Scientist* Vo. 89 (2001): 406–12.

Ploegh, Hidde. "Viral Strategies of Immune Evasion." *Science* Vol. 280 (1998): 248–253.

Jones, Philip S. "Strategies for Antiviral Drug Discovery." *Antiviral Chemistry and Chemotherapy* Vol. 9.4 (1998): 283–302.

Bernstein, Jack M. *Antiviral Chemotherapy: General Overview.* Dayton, OH: Wright State University School of Medicine, Division of Infectious Diseases, 2000.

Page, Roderic D. M., and Edward C. Holmes. *Molecular Evolution.* Boston, MA: Blackwell Science, 1988.

Collier, Leslie, and John Oxford. *Human Virology.* Oxford, England: Oxford University Press, 2000.

Yanick, P. "Immune System Protection against Bioterrorism." *Townsend Letter for Doctors & Patients,* Dec., 2001.

Cody, V., et al. *Plant Flavonoids in Biology and Medicine. Biochemical, Cellular, and Molecular Properties* New York: Alan R. Liss, 1988.

Yanick, P. "Meridian/Organ Nutraceutic Resonant Complexes: New Hope for Chronically-Sick Individuals." *Townsend Letter for Doctors & Patients,* May, 2000.

Yanick, P. "Boosting Nutrient Uptake in Chronic Illness." *Townsend Letter for Doctors & Patients,* Dec., 2000.

Yanick, P. "Food Supplement Benefits and Risks in Carcinogenesis: Part I." *Townsend Letter for Doctors & Patients.* Oct., 2001.

Borchers, A. T., et al. "Mushrooms, Tumors, and Immunity." *Proceedings of the Society of Experimental Biological Medicine* Vol. 4 (1999): 282–93.

Kabara, J. J., et al. "Fatty Acids and Derivatives as Antimicrobial Agents." *Antimicrobial Agents and Chemotherapy* (1992): 23–28.

Kabara, J. J. "Toxicological, Bacteriocidal and Fungicidal Properties of Fatty Acids and Some Derivatives." *JAOCS* Vol. 56 (1979): 760.

Hierholzer, J. C., and Kabara, J. J. "In Vitro Effects of Monolaurin Compounds on Enveloped RNA and DNA Viruses." *J. Food Safety* Vol. 4 (1982): 1–12.

Enig, M. G. *Coconut Oil: An Anti-bacterial, Anti-viral Ingredient for Food, Nutrition and Health.* Manila, Philippines: AVOC Luric Symposium, 1997.

McTaggert, L. *The Field: The Quest for the Secret Force of the Universe.* New York: Harper Collins, 2001.

Popp, A. F. *Biophotonen.* Heidelberg, Germany: Schriftenreihe Krebsgeschehen, 1984.

Verastegui, M. Angeles, et al. "Antimicrobial Activity of Extracts of Three Major Plants of the Chichuahuan Desert." *J of Enthopharmacology* Vol. 52 (1996): 175–77.

Brinker, F. "Larrea tridentata." *British J of Phytotherapy* Vol. 3.1. (1994): 10–30.

Kawagishi, H., et al. "Herinacines A,B,C, Strong Stimulators of Nerve Growth Factor from the Mushroom *Hericium.*" *Tetrahedron Letters* Vol. 32 (1991): 4561–64.

Kawagishi, H., et al: "Herinacines A,B,C, Strong Stimulators of Nerve Growth Factor from the Mushroom *Hericium.*" *Tetrahedron Letters* Vol. 35.10 (1994): 1569–72.

Scott, D. W., and W. L. Scott. *The Extremely Unfortunate Skull Valley Incident.* Chelmsford, Canada: Chelmsford Publishers, 2001.

Scott, D. W., and W. L. Scott. *The Brucellosis Triangle.* Chelmsford, Canada: Chemsford Publishers, 1998.

Lo, S. "Pathogenic Mycoplasma." US Patent 5,242,820, issued 9–7–93.

World Health Organization. *Report on the Panel on Food and Agriculture.* Geneva, Switzerland: World Health Organization, 1992.

Bell, I. R "A Time-Dependent Sensitization in Environmental Illness: A Pharmacologic Model." The Eleventh International Symposium on Man and His Environment in Health and Disease.1993. November 29, 2002 http://www.aehf.com/articles/1993symp.html.

Bell, I. R., et al. "An Olfactory-limbic Model of Multiple Chemical Sensitivity Syndrome." *Biological Psychiatry* Vol. 32 (1992): 218–242.

Lorig, T., et al. "EEG Activity during Administration of Low-concentration Odors." *Bulletin of Psychonomic Science* Vol. 28 (1990): 405–8.

Gilbert, M. E. "Neurotoxicants and Limbic Kindling." In R. L. Isaacs and K. F. Jensen, Eds., *The Vulnerable Brain and Environmental Risks,* Vol. I. New York: Plenum Press.1992.

Constantini, A. V. " The Fungal/Mycotoxin Etiology of Atherosclerosis and Hyperlipidemia." 1993. The Eleventh International Symposium on Man and His Environment in Health and Disease. November 29, 2002 http://www.aehf.com/articles/1993symp.html.

Richard, J. L. "In G. E. Bray and D. H. Ryan, Eds. *Mycotoxins, Cancer, and Health.* Baton-Rouge, LA: Louisiana State University Press, 1991.

Delincee, H., and B. Pool-Aobel. "Genotoxic Properties of 2–dodecycobutanone, a Compound Formed by Irradiation of Food Containing Fat." *Radiation Physics and Chemistry* Vol. 52 (1988): 39–42.

Le Tellier, P. R., and W. W. Mawar. "2–alkalcyclobutanones from the Radiolysis of Triglycerides." *Lipids* Vol. 7 (1972): 76–76.

Delincee, H., et al. "Genotoxicity of 2–alkalcyclobutanones Markers for Irradiation Treatment in Fat-Containing Food. A paper presented at the 12th International Meeting on Radiation Processing. Avignon, France: March 25–30, 2001.

Miller, C. S. "Toxicology and Industrial Health." *New Engl. J. Med.* 335.2A (1992):1498–1504.

Chapter 9. The Brain: Our QEF Regenerator

Enig, M. G. "Coconut, in Support of Good Health in the 21st Century." *36th Asian Pacific Coconut Community,* 1999.

Enig, M. G. *Coronary Heart Disease: The Dietary Sense and Nonsense.* London, England: Janus Publishing, 1993.

Fife, B. *The Miracles of Coconut Oil.* Colorado Springs, CO: Healthwise. 2000.

Kabara. J. J., et al. "Fatty Acids and Derivatives as Antimicrobial Agents." *Antimicrobial Agents and Chemotherapy* (1992): 23–28.

Kabara. J. J. "Toxicological, Bacteriocidal and Fungicidal Properties of Fatty Acids and Some Derivatives." *JAOCS* Vol. 56 (1979): 760.

Hierholzer, J. C., and Kabra J. J. "In Vitro Effects of Monolaurin Compounds on Enveloped RNA and DNA Viruses. *J. Food Safety* Vol 4 (1982): 1–12.

Enig, M. G. *Coconut Oil: An Anti-bacterial, Anti-viral Ingredient for Food, Nutrition and Health.* Manila, Philippines: AVOC Luric Symposium, 1997.

Yanick, P. "Immune System Protection against Bioterrorism." *Townsend Letter for Doctors & Patients,* Dec., 2001.

Yanick, P. "Novel Anti-viral Strategies." *Townsend Letter for Doctors & Patients,* Feb./March, 2002.

Loviselli, A., et al. "Low Levels of Dehydroepiandrosterone Sulfate in Adult Males with Insulin-Dependent Diabetes Mellitus. *Minerva Endocrinology* Vol. 19 (1994): 113–119.

Van Vollenhoven, R. F., et al. "An Open Study of Dehydroepiandrosterone in Systemic Lupus Erthematosus." *Arthritis Rheum* Vol. 37 (1994):1305–1310.

Jacobson, M., et al. "Decreased Serum Dehydroepiandrosterone Is Associated with an Increased Progression of Human Immunodeficiency Virus Infection in Men with CD4 Cell Counts of 200–499." *Journal of Infectious Diseases,* Vol. 164.5 (1991): 864 (5).

Ebeling, P., et al. "Physiological Importance of Dehydroepiandrosterone." *The Lancet* Vol. 343 (1994): 1479.

Fava, M., et al. "Dehydroepiandrosterone-Sulfate/Cortisol Ratio in Panic Disorder. *Psychiatry Res.* Vol. 28 (1989): 345–350.

Atschule, M., and J. Kitay. *McLead Hospital Pineal Research Collections,* 1940.

Beck-Friis, J., et al. "Serum Melatonin in Relation to Clinical Variables in Patients with Major Depressive Disorder and a Hypothesis of a Low Melatonin Syndrome." *Acta Psychiatrica Scandinavia* Vol. 71(1985): 319–30.

Cavallo, A., et al. "Melatonin Circadian Rhythm in Childhood Depression." *Journal of the American Academy of Child and Adolescent Psychiatry* Vol. 26.3 (1987): 395–99.

Selkoe, D.J. "Amyloid Protein and Alzheimer's Disease." *Scientific American* Vol. 4 (1993): 54–58.

Linder, M.E., and A. G. Gilman. "G Proteins." *Scientific American,* 1993.

Pischinger, A. *Matrix and Matrix Regulation.* Brussels, Belgium: Haug Publishers, 1991.

Kartner, N., and V. Ling. "Multidrug Resistance in Cancer." *Scientific American,* 1993.

Carskadon, M.A., and C. Acebo. "Parental Reports of Seasonal Mood and Behavior Changes in Children." *Journal of the American Academy of Child and Adolescent Psychiatry* Vol. 32.2 (1993): 246.

Wehr, T. A. "The Durations of Human Melatonin Secretion and Sleep Respond to the Changes in Daylength (Photoperiod)." *Journal of Clinical Endocrinology and Metabolism* Vol. 73.6 (1991): 1276–80.

Krauchi, K., et al. "The Relationship of Affective Disorder State to Dietary Preference: Winter Depression and Light Therapy as a Model." *Journal of Affective Disorders* Vol. 20 (1990): 43–53.

Rao, M. L., et al. "The Influence of Phototherapy on Serotonin and Melatonin in Non-seasonal Depression. *Pharmacopsychiatry* Vol. 23 (1990): 155–58.

Anton-Tay, F. "On the Effect of Melatonin upon Human Brain: Its Possible Therapeutic Implications." *Life Sciences* Vol. 10 (1971): 841–50.

Demisch, L. *Clinical Pharmacology of Melatonin Regulation.* Boca Raton, FL: CRC Press, 1993.

Wilson, B. W., C. Wright, and L. E. Anderson. "Evidence for an Effect of ELF Electromagnetic Fields on Human Pineal Gland Function." *Journal of Pineal Research* Vol. 9 (1990): 259–69.

Semm, P., et al. "Effects of an Earth-Strength Magnetic Field on Electrical Activity of Pineal Cells." *Nature* Vol. 288 (1980): 607–8.

Wilson, B. W., et al. "Neuroendocrine Mediated Effects of Electromagnetic-Field Exposure: Possible Role of the Pineal Gland." *Life Sciences* Vol. 45 (1985): 1319–32.

"Correlation Between Heart Attacks and Magnetic Activity." *Nature* Vol. 277 (1994): 646–48.

Dubbels, R., et al. "Melatonin Determination with a Newly Developed ELISA System: Inter-individual Differences in the Response of the Human Pineal Gland to Magnetic Fields." In G. J. Maestroni, A. Conti, and R. J. Reiter, Eds. *Advances in Pineal Research*, Vol. 7. London: John Libbey and Co., 1994.

Chapter 10. Quantum Foods

Doll, R., et al. "The Causes of Cancer." *J Nat Cancer Institute* Vol. 66: (1981): 1191.

World Cancer Research Fund. "Food, Nutrition and the Prevention of Cancer. A Global Perspective." Washington, D.C.: American Institute for Cancer Research, 1997.

Cummings, J. H., et al. "Diet and the Prevention of Cancer." *BMJ* Vol. 317 (1998): 1636–40.

Houston, M. D., and J. S. Strupp. "Prevention and Treatment of Cancer: Is the Cure in the Produce Aisle?" *JAMA* Vol. 3.3 (2000): 27–30.

Block J. B., and S. Evans. "Clinical Evidence Supporting Cancer Risk Reduction with Antioxidants and Implications for Diets and Supplements." *JAMA*. Vol. 3.3 (2000): 6–16.

Jensen, B., and M. Anderson. *Empty Harvest*. Garden City Park, New York.: Avery, 1990.

"Veggie Nutrients Dip in Tests." *Omaha World-Herald*, January 29,2000: 6.

Finely, J., et al. "Selenium Content of Foods Purchased in North Dakota." *Nutr. Res.* Vol. 16 (1996): 723–28.

Hu, J., et al. "Risk Factors for Oesophageal Cancer in Northeast China." *Int J Cancer* Vol. 57 (1994): 38–46.

Haung, M. T., et al. "Inhibition of Skin Tumorgenesis by Rosemary and Its Constituents Carnosol and Ursolic Acid." *Cancer Research* Vol. 54 (1994): 701–8.

Steinmetz, K. A., et al. "Vegetables, Fruit, and Cancer Prevention: A Review." *J Am Diet Association* Vol. 96 (1996): 27–37.

Winter, et al. *Chemicals in the Human Food Chain*. Basel, Germany: Van Nostrand Reinhold, 1990.

World Health Organization. *Report on the Panel on Food and Agriculture*. Geneva, Switzerland: World Health Organization, 1992.

Minchin, R. F., et al. Role of Acetylation in Colorectal Cancer. *Mutation Research* Vol. 290 (1993.): 35–42.

Sinha, R., et al. "High Concentrations of the Carcinogen 2–amino-1–methel-6–phenykunudazi Occur in Chicken but Are Dependent on the Cooking Method." *Cancer Res* Vol. 55 (1996): 4516–19.

Snyderwibe, E. G. "Some Perspective on the Nutritional Aspects of Breast Cancer Research. Food Derived HCAs as Etiologic Agents in Human Mammary Cancer." *Cancer* Vol. 74 (1994): 977–94.

Sacarello, H. L. A. *Handbook of Hazardous Materials*. Washington, DC: Lewis Publishers, 1994.

See, D. *Journal of the American Nutraceutical Association* Vol. 2.1 (1996): 25–41.

Yanick, P. "Meridian/Organ Nutraceutic Resonant Complexes: New Hope for Chronically-Sick Individuals." *Townsend Letter for Doctors & Patients*, May, 2000, 136–39.

Yanick, P. "Boosting Nutrient Uptake in Chronic Illness." *Townsend Letter for Doctors & Patients*, December 2000.

Marshall, R. *Ten Secrets You May Not Know*. Round Rock, TX: Premier Research Labs, 2001.

Khachik, F., et al. "Distribution, Bioavailability and Metabolism of Carotenoids in Humans." In W. R. Bidlack, S. T. Omaye, et al, Eds. *Phytochemicals: A New Paradigm*. Basel, Germany: Technomic Pub, Inc., 1998.

Kuhlmann, M. K., et al. "Reduction of Cisplatinin Toxicity in Cultured Renal Tubular Cells by the Bioflavonoid Quercitin." *Arch Toxicology* Vol. 72 (1998): 536–40.

Venkatesan, N. "Curcumin Attenuation of Acute Adriamycin Myocardial Toxicity in Rats." *Br. J Pharm.* Vol. 124 (1998): 425–27.

Furr, H. C., et al. "Intestinal Absorption and Tissue Distribution of Carotenoids." *Nutr Biochemistry* Vol. 8 (1997): 364–77.

Ferriola, P. C., et al. "Protein Kinase C Inhibition by Plant Flavonoids." *Biochem Pharmacol.* Vol. 38 (1989): 1617–24.

Agullo, G., et al. "Relationship between Structure and Inhibition of Phosphotidylinositol 3–kinase: a Comparison with Tyrosine Kinase and Protein Kinase C Inhibition." *Biochem pharmacology* Vol. 53 (1997): 1649–57.

Hoffman, J., et al. "Enhancement of the Antiproliferative Effect of Cis-damminedichloroplatinum (II) and Nitrogen Mustard by Inhibitors of Protein Kinase C." *Int J Cancer* Vol. 42 (1998): 382–88.

Scambia, G., et al. "Inhibitory Effect of Quercitin on Primary Ovarian and Endometrial Cancers and Synergistic Activity with Cis-damminedichloroplatinum (II)." *Gyn Oncology* Vol.45 (1992): 13–19.

Wang, Z., et al. "Mammary Cancer Promotion and MAPK Activation Associated with Consumption of a Corn Oil-based High Fat Diet." *Nutr Cancer* Vol. 34: (1999): 140–46.

Hurston, S. D., et al. "Types of Dietary Fat and the Incidence of Cancer at Five Sites." *Prev Med.* Vol. 9 (1990): 242–53.

Yanick, P. *A Professional's Guidebook to Quantum Medicine*. American Academy of Quantum Medicine, 2001.

Vojdani, A., et al. "New Evidence for the Antioxidant Properties of Vitamin C." *Intern Soc of Prev Oncology* Vol. 24.6 (2000): 508–523.

Vojdani, A., and G. Namatalla. "Enhancement of NK Cytoxic Activity by Vitamin C in Pure and Augmented Formulations." *J Nutr Envirn Medicine* Vol. 7 (1997): 187–95.

Havlick, H. D. "Functional Foods: Science or Marketing?" *JAMA* Vol. 4.1 (2001): 9–10.

Macleod, R. L., et al. "Inhibition of Intestinal Secretion by Rice." *Lancet* (1995): 90–92.

Gates, J. R., et al. "Association of Dietary Factors and Selected Plasma Variables with Sex-hormone-binding Globulin in Rural Chinese Women." *Am J Clin Nutrition* Vol. 36 (1996): 22–31.

Blobel, G., et al. "Metal Ion Chaperone Function of the Soluble Cu(I) Receptor Axis." *Science* Vol. 278 (1997): 853–56.

Yanick, P. "Dietary and Lifestyle Influences on Cochlear Disorders and Biochemical Status: A Twelve-month Study." *Journal of Applied Nutrition* Vol. 40, no. 2, (1988).

Gushleff, B. W. "The Role of Novel Phyto-Estrogen and Progestogen Therapy in the Menopausal Patient." *Informedica* Vol. 314 (1986): 205.

Yanick, P. "Physiological-Chemical Assessment of Undernutrition." *Townsend Letter for Doctors*, July, 1988.

Yanick, P. "Biomolecular Nutrition and the GI Tract." *Townsend Letter for Doctors*, Dec. ,1993.

Adibi, S., E. Phillips. "Evidence for Greater Absorption of Amino Acids from Peptide than from Free Form in Human Intestine." *Clin Research* Vol. 16 (1968): 446.

Craft, I. L., et al. "Absorption and Malabsorption of Glycine and Glycine Peptides in Man." *Gut* Vol. 9 (1968): 425–437.

Adibi, S.A., M. R. Fogel, and R. M. Agrawal. "Comparison of Free Amino Acid and Dipeptide Absorption in the Jejunum of Sprue Patients." *Gastroenterology* Vol. 67 (1974): 586–591.

Reicht, G., W. Petritsch, A. Eherer, et al. "Jejunal Protein Absorption of Whey Protein and Its Hydrolysate." *JPEN* Vol. 16 (1992): 25S.

Neredith J. W., J. A. Ditesheim, and G. P. Zaloga. "Visceral Protein Levels in Trauma Patients Are Greater with Peptide Diet than Intact Protein Diet." *J Trauma* Vol 30 (1990): 825–829.

Gardner, M.G. "Intestinal Assimilation of Intact Peptides and Proteins from the Diet-A Neglected Field." *Biol Review* Vol. 59 (1984): 289–331.

Boullin, D.J., R. F. Crampton, C. E. Heading , et al. "Intestinal Absorption of Dipeptides Containing Glycine, Phenylalanine, Proline, B-alanine, or Histidine in the Rat." *Clinical Science Molecular Medicine* Vol. 45 (1973): 849–858.

Gardner, M.G. "Absorption of Intact Peptides: Studies on Transport of Protein Digest and Dipeptides across Rat Small Intestine *in Vitro.*" *Q J Exp Physiol* Vol. 67 (1982): 629–637.

Kontessis, P., S. Jones, R. Dodds, et al. "Renal, Metabolic and Hormonal Responses to Ingestion of Animal and Vegetable Proteins." *Kidney Int* Vol. 38 (1990): 136–144.

Silk, D.B.A., P. D. Fairclough, M. L. Clark, et al. "Use of a Peptide Rather than Free Amino Nitrogen Source in Chemically Defined 'Elemental' Diets." *JPEN* Vol. 4 (1980): 548–553.

Keohane P.P., G. K. Grimble, B. Brown, et al. "Influence of Protein Composition and Hydrolysis Method on Intestinal Absorption of Protein in Man." *Gut* Vol. 26 (1985): 907–913.

Webb, K.E. "Amino Acid and Peptide Absorption from the Gastrointestinal Tract. *Federation Proceeding* Vol. 45 (1986): 2268–2271.

Amoss, M., J. Rivier, R. Guillemin. "Release of Gonadotropins by Oral Administration of Synthetic LRF or a Tripeptide Fragment of LRF." *J Clin Endocrinology Metab* Vol. 35 (1972): 175–177.

Bowers, C. Y., A. V. Schally, F. Enzmann, F., et al. "Porcine Thyrotrophin Releasing Hormone Is (Pyro)Glu-His-Pro(NH2)." *Endocrinology* Vol. 86 (1970): 1143–1153.

Gardner, M.L.G. "Entry of Peptides of Dietary Origin into the Circulation." *Nutr Health* Vol. 2 (1983): 163–171.

Adibi, S. A. "Intestinal Absorption of Dipeptides in Man: Relative Importance of Hydrolysis and Intact Absorption." *J Clin Invest* Vol 50 (1971): 2266–2275.

Newey, H., and D. H. Smyth, "The Intestinal Absorption of Some Dipeptides." *J Physiol* Vol. 145 (1959): 48–56.

Cody, V., et al. *Plant Flavonoids in Biology and Medicine II.* New York: Alan R Liss, 1988.

Higashi K. O. "Propolis Extracts Are Effective against Trypanosome Cruzi and Have an Impact on Its Interaction with Cells." *J Ethnopharmacology* Vol. 8.4 (1994): 149–55.

Rao, C. V., et al. "Effect of Caffeic Acid Esters on Carcinogen-induced Mutagenecity and Human Colon Adenocarcinoma Cell Growth." *Chemical and Biological Interactions* Vol. 84 (1992): 277–90.

Pariza, M. "CLA Reduces Body Fat." *FASEB Journal* Vol. 10 (1996): A3227.

Blankson, H., et al. "CLA Reduces Body Fat Mass in Obese and Overweight Humans." *J Nutrition* Vol. 130 (2000): 2943–8.

Ip, C., et al. "Mammary Cancer Prevention by CLA." *Cancer Research* Vol. 51.22 (1991): 6118–24.

Parodi, P. W. "Cow's Milk Components as Potential Anticarcinogenic." *J Nutr* Vol. 127 (1997): 1055–60.

Wahke, et al. "Fatty Acids and Endothelial Cell Function: Regulation of Adhesion Molecule and Redox Enzyme Expression." *Curr Opin Clin Nutr Metab Care* Vol. 2.2 (1999): 109–15.

Chapter 11. The Quantum Energy Diet

Campbell, T. C. "A Plant-Enriched Diet and Long-term Health, Particularly in Reference to China." Paper presented at the Second International Symposium on Horticulture and Human Health, Alexandria, VA: November 4, 1989.

Campbell, T. C. et al., "China: From Diseases of Poverty to Diseases of Affluence. Policy Implications of the Epidemiological Transition." Paper part of NIH Grant 5R01CA33638. Bethesda, MD: National Institutes of Health, 1990.

Ornish, D., et al., "Can Lifestyle Changes Reverse Coronary Heart Disease? (The Life-style Heart Trial)." *The Lancet* Vol. 336 (1990): 129–133.

Ellis, F. R., et al., "Incidence of Osteoporosis in Vegetarians and Ommivores." *American Journal of Clinical Nutrition* Vol. 6 (1972): 555–558.

Ihle, B. U., et al., "The Effect of Protein Restriction on the Progression of Renal Insufficiency." *New England Journal of Medicine* Vol. 321 (1989): 1773–1777.

Walford, R. "The Clinical Promise of Diet Restriction." *Geriatrics* Vol. 45 (1990): 81–87.

Brenner, B. M., et al., "Dietary Protein Intake and the Progressive Nature of Kidney Disease." *New England Journal of Medicine* Vol. 307 (1982): 652–659.

Young, V. R., and P. L. Pellett. "Protein Intake and Requirements with Reference to Diet and Health." *American Journal of Clinical Nutrition* Vol. 45 (1987):1323–1343.

Irwin, I. M., and D. M. Hegsted. "A Conspectus of Research on Protein Requirements of Man." *The Journal of Nutrition* Vol. 101 (1971): 385–430.

Walford, Roy L. *Maximum Lifespan.* New York: Norton & Co., 1983.

Walford, Roy L. *The One Hundred and Twenty Year Diet: How to Double Your Vital Years.* New York: Simon & Schuster, 1987.

McCay, C.M., M. F. Crowell, and L. A. Maynard. "The Effect of Retarded Growth upon the Length of Life Span and upon the Ultimate Body Size." *J. Nutrition* Vol. 10 (1935):63–79.

Masoro, E. J. "Food Restriction in Rodents: An Evaluation of Its Role in the Study of Aging." *J. Gerontology* Vol. 43 (1988): B59–B64.

Weindruch, R., and R. L. Walford. *The Retardation of Aging and Disease by Dietary Restriction.* Springfield, IL: Charles C Thomas, 1988.

Chvapil, M., and Z. Hruza. "The Influence of Aging and Undernutrition on Chemical Contractility and Relaxation of Collagen Fibers in Rats." *Gerontologia* Vol. 3 (1959): 241–52.

Ingram, D. K., R. Weindruch, E. L. Spangler, et al. "Dietary Restriction Benefits Learning and Motor Performance of Aged Mice." *J. Gerontology* Vol 42 (1987): 78–81.

Berg, B. N., and H. S. Simms. "Nutrition and Longevity in the Rats. II. Longevity and Onset of Disease with Different Levels of Food Intake." *J. Nutrition* Vol. 71 (1960): 255–63.

Yu, B. P., E. J. Masoro, I. Murata, et al. "Life Span Study of SPF Fischer: 344 Male Rats Fed *Ad Libitum* or Restricted Diets: Longevity, Growth, Lean Body Mass and Disease." *J Gerontology* Vol. 37 (1982):130–141.

McCay, Clive M., et al. "The Life Span of Rats on a Restricted Diet." *Journal of Nutrition* Vol. 18 (1939):1–25.

McCay, Clive M. "Effect of Restricted Feeding upon Aging and Chronic Disease in Rats and Dogs." *American Journal of Public Health* Vol. 37 (1947): 521.

Mazess, R. B., and W. Mather. "Bone Mineral Content of North Alaskan Eskimos." *American Journal of Clinical Nutrition* Vol. 27 (1974): 916–925.

Williams, Clyde. "Diet and Endurance Fitness." *American Journal of Clinical Nutrition* Vol. 49 (1989): 1077–1083.

Masoro, E. J., I. Shimokawa, and B. P. Yu. "Retardation of Aging Process in Rats by Food Restriction." *Ann. NY Acad. Sci.* Vol. 621 (1991): 337–52.

Yu, B. P. "Food Restriction Research: Past and Present Status." *Rev. Biol. Res. Aging* Vol. 4 (1990): 349–71.

Jung, L. K. L., M. A. Palladino, S. Calvano, et al. "Effect of Calorie Restriction on the Production and Responsiveness to Interleukin-2 in (NZBXZW) f-1 Mice." *Clinical Immunology Immunopathology* Vol. 25(1982): 295–301.

Perpaoli, W., A. Dall'ara, E. Pedrinis, and W. Regelson. "The Pineal Control of Aging. The Effects of Melatonin and Pineal Grafting on the Survival of Older Mice." *Ann. NY Acad. Sci.* Vol. 621 (1991): 291–313.

Anisimov, V. N., L. A. Bondarenko, V. K. Khavinson, and V. G. Morozov. "The Pineal Peptides: Interaction with Indoles and the Role in Aging and Cancer." *Neuroendocrinology. Letter* Vol. 11 (1989): 235.

Walker, R. F., K. M. McMahon, and E. B. Pivorun. "Pineal Gland Structure and Respiration as Affected by Age and Hypocaloric Diet." *Exp. Gerontology* Vol. 13 (1978): 91–99.

Stokkan, K. A., R. J. Reiter, K. O. Nonaka, et al. "Food Restriction Retards Aging of the Pineal Gland." *Brain Research* Vol. 545 (1991): 66–72.

Everitt, A. V. "Food Intake, Growth and the Aging of Collagen in Rat Tail Tendon." *Gerontologia* Vol. 17 (1971): 98–104.

Deyl, Z., M. Juricova, J. Rosmus, and M. Adam. "The Effect of Food Deprivation on Collagen Accumulation." *Exp. Gerontology* Vol. 6 (1971): 383–90.

Czeisler, C., et al. "Suppression of Melatonin Secretion in Some Blind Patients by Exposure to Bright Light." *N England J Med* Vol. 332 (1995): 6–11.

Rieter, R. J., and J. Robinson. "Creating a Melatonin-Friendly Lifestyle." *The Natural Way.* March–April, 1996.

Huether, G., B. Poeggeler, A. Reimer, and A. George. "Effect of Tryptophan Administration on Circulating Melatonin Levels in Chicks and Rats: Evidence for Stimulation of Melatonin Synthesis and Release in the Gastrointestinal Tract." *Life Sciences* Vol. 51 (1992): 945–953.

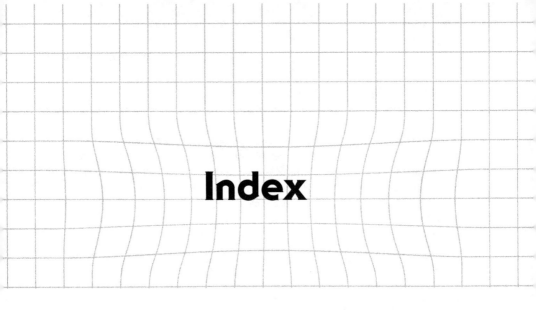

Index